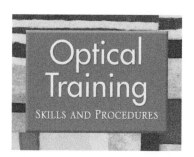

Optical Training
SKILLS AND PROCEDURES

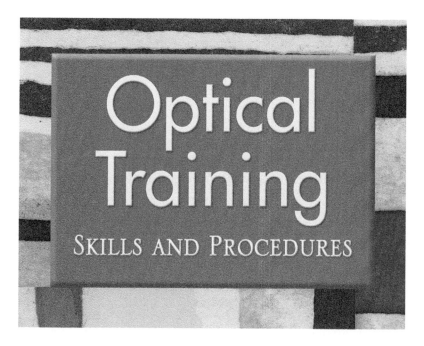

Optical Training

SKILLS AND PROCEDURES

Davey M. Wooton, ABOC

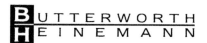

BUTTERWORTH
HEINEMANN

An Imprint of Elsevier Science

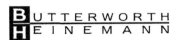

An Imprint of Elsevier Science

11830 Westline Industrial Drive
St. Louis, Missouri 63146

OPTICAL TRAINING: SKILLS AND PROCEDURES   ISBN 0-7506-7477-6
Copyright © 2003, Elsevier Science (USA). All rights reserved.

Library of Congress Cataloging-in-Publication Data

Wooton, Davey.
  Basic optical knowledge: the working manual for new opticians/Davey Wooton.
    p. cm.
  ISBN 0-7506-7477-6 (alk. paper)
    1. Opticians–Handbooks, manuals, etc. 2. Physiological optics–Handbooks, manuals, etc. I. Title.

RE952.9.W66 2003
617.7'5–dc21

                                                                          2003048709

Publishing Director: Linda Duncan
Managing Editor: Christie Hart
Project Manager: Joy Moore
Senior Book Designer: Amy Buxton

PREFACE

I am an American Board of Opticianry (ABO)-certified optician with 10 years' experience as a laboratory technician, dispensing optician, ophthalmic technician, and assistant manager. I have worked in different locations in three states, and I have found that there is always one common problem. It is difficult to find enough experienced people in this field to fill the needed positions. Normally, the persons hired have no optical experience at all. It takes a lot of energy and time to train them and to give them all of the knowledge required to perform the job with confidence and efficiency.

Many textbooks and tools are available to help the optician become certified and achieve higher degrees of certification. All of these textbooks and tools are good, but they all are designed assuming the optician already has a *basic* working knowledge of optics. The problem still remains—providing the optician with the basic working knowledge in a way that is easy to understand and is not overwhelming.

I have developed a training schedule and handbook that explain all of the basics in a simplified manner. My handbook prepares anyone who has no knowledge of optics to be able to perform his or her job duties within a reasonable amount of time without being overwhelming. He or she should be able to perform the day-to-day duties with a solid foundation of the necessary information. It will also help current opticians go back and review the basics. The handbook is also designed to aid in assessing the level of knowledge of an experienced optician who is new to the company.

This handbook is intended for the optician who has no previous exposure to optical. Each topic covered in the book can be expanded on greatly. The purpose of the book is to educate the optician without overwhelming him or her. We have to keep this in mind while training the new optician. We have more experience and knowledge. It is easy to start delving into more depth but this only confuses and overwhelms him or her. We have to pull ourselves back at times and keep to the basics and make sure that the optician learns and comprehends the material. This will lay the foundation of core information the optician needs to perform his or her job well. There will be time in the future to educate the optician further and prepare him or her for certification.

Davey Wooton

CONTENTS

Level 3 Optician Apprentice *66*

Level 4 Optician *93*

Answers to Assessments *107*

Index *110*

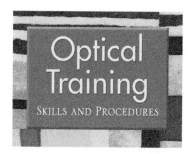

INTRODUCTION

TASK SCHEDULE FOR NEW OPTICIANS AND NEW HIRES

The following schedule was designed to guide the new optician and the trainer at a steady pace without overwhelming them. The schedule can also be used to assess the level of knowledge of an experienced optician that is a new hire to the company. The manual is written in a plain, simple definition form. The assessments are at the end of each level.

I have tried to include all the information that is necessary to carry out the daily duties of an optician. The subject of optics is more complicated. Further study of optics is strongly encouraged. It can only help you become a better and more confident optician. A few of the selections recommended for reading are *Professional Dispensing for Opticianry* (Opticians Association of America Staff, Butterworth-Heinemann, 1996), *Understanding Lens Surfacing* (CW Brooks, Butterworth-Heinemann, 1992), and *Contact Lenses: Procedures and Techniques* (GE Lowther, C Snyder, Butterworth-Heinemann, 1992).

TASK OUTLINE FOR NEW OPTICIANS AND NEW HIRES

This is an overall view of each task to be mastered.

TASKS TO MASTER

Level 1 New Hire (Follow Trainer)

Become acquainted with fellow staff members	
Learn office procedure and policy	
Learn how to handle third-party accounts and payments	
Learn how to read price sheets	
Learn how to use the time clock and keep track of hours	
Read assigned material: *Basic Job Duties*	
Read assigned material: *Common Office Equipment*	
Read assigned material: *Phone Protocol*	
Read assigned material: *Laboratory Process*	
Read assigned material: *Doctors and Technicians*	
Complete *Level 1 Assessment*	

Level 2 Office Assistant (Work with Supervision)

Familiarize yourself with frame lines carried in your office	
Start answering phones	
Be able to quote prices	
Read assigned material: *Making Appointments*	
Read assigned material: *The Eye*	
Read assigned material: *Eye Conditions*	
Read assigned material: *Light and Refraction*	
Read assigned material: *Frames*	
Read assigned material: *Adjustments*	
Read assigned material: *Lenses*	
Read assigned material: *Lens Coatings and Extras*	
Read assigned material: *Basic Written Contact Lens Prescription*	
Read assigned material: *Contact Lenses*	
Complete *Level 2 Assessment*	

Level 3 Optician Apprentice (Work with Light Supervision)

Read assigned material: *More About Lenses*	
Read assigned material: *Choosing Lenses*	
Read assigned material: *Face Shapes*	
Read assigned material: *Frame Styling*	
Read assigned material: *Taking Measurements*	
Read assigned material: *Lensometer*	
Read assigned material: *Transposing*	
Complete *Level 3 Assessment*	

Level 4 Optician (Work Without Supervision)

Read assigned material: *Job Orders and Sales*	
Read assigned material: *Dispensing Glasses*	
Read assigned material: *Dispensing Contact Lenses*	
Read assigned material: *Troubleshooting*	
Read assigned material: *Verifying Glasses*	
Complete *Level 4 Assessment*	

With each level, the optician's knowledge and confidence should be growing.

THE MANUAL

If you are the trainer, you should read the manual and assessments before the hire date of the new optician. This will help you become familiar with the material that is covered and brush up on your skills. Knowing what the new optician will be reading helps you understand what he or she is going through. You will be better prepared to answer any questions he or she may have, having already reviewed the material.

Other opticians in your office should review the manual so that everyone is on the same page when the new optician is hired. You may enlist the help of fellow opticians when training the new optician. These other opticians will have an understanding of what the new optician is learning and will be better informed to answer questions. It allows them to brush up their skills, and it will help everyone work more like a united team.

The manual should be used as a guide, and the material should be tailored to the practical use for your office. Some information may not apply, such as contact lens care, laboratory work, or having a doctor on staff. Although you may not have these operations in effect at your location, knowing how they work and what is involved in the different areas can help you and your opticians do a better job.

You will find that much of the information in the manual is repeated. I believe that repetition of information is one of the best teachers. It provides reinforcement of material and makes learning easier.

If the new hire has experience, ask him or her to take the assessments so that you can identify his or her level of knowledge. The new hire may continue reading the manual if he or she needs to brush up on skills or needs learn more. The manual can also be used as a primer for certification.

PREPARING THE OPTICIAN

If possible, one person should be designated to train the new optician. This will create more consistency in the learning process.

Prepare the optician for work by stating what is expected of him or her. Let the new hire know the standards your office upholds. The optician will feel more comfortable knowing what goals he or she is expected to achieve. In addition, when everyone in the office is held to the same standards, it creates more of a teamwork atmosphere. Everyone understands that you are all striving for the same goal and you are all held accountable for your actions.

You should follow the schedule as much as possible. Some tasks may need to be spread out because of the optician's or the trainer's work schedule. This is fine as long as the optician works on the information in order. If the information seems to be thrown at him or her out of sequence, it will cause confusion and misunderstandings.

Assure the optician that the assessments are *not* a pass or fail system. They are used simply to find the optician's strengths and to identify areas which may need more concentration. Some information is more difficult to grasp, especially information about lenses and lens design. It may be necessary to repeat these areas. The assessments are your way of evaluating the optician's progress.

STAFF INTRODUCTIONS

The introductions to fellow staff members are important for you and the optician. They allow you to show how each person on staff is important. Each member makes his or her own contribution to making your office run smoothly. The new optician has a chance to learn about future job opportunities that are available with your company. Fellow employees also get a chance to welcome the new staff member and feel like they are important enough to be introduced to "the new guy." It makes everyone feel important, because everyone *is* important.

The introductions should be as personal as possible. For instance, they should not be made by passing someone and saying, "Oh yeah, that's so-and-so. This is the new guy." Each employee should be sought out. You should stand with both employees and properly introduce them to each other. "Hello Bob! This is Jane, our newest team member. Jane, this is Bob. He is our laboratory technician. He makes all the glasses that come through here. If you ever have a question about lenses or glasses in general, come see him. You can trust he knows what he's talking about. Bob, tell Jane a little about your experience and background." An introduction such as this does many things for the new optician and the current employee.

1. It helps the new optician know who everyone is and the various job duties.
2. It establishes credibility of the current employee to the new optician.
3. It makes the current employee feel validated. Everyone loves to talk about himself or herself and show off a little bit of his or her knowledge.
4. It opens the lines of communication between the new and current employees.

You may want to brag a little about the current employee. It makes him or her feel valuable. You should set personal feelings aside and think about each employee's contribution to the office. The new employee will also know that if he or she performs well, you will brag about him or her too.

A personal introduction is important; however, some people may not take it seriously. It may seem like a small thing to do, but it will create more of a team atmosphere for you and the employees. If a person feels valued and respected, he or she will be a hard-working, loyal employee.

ROLE-PLAYING

Role-playing is a tool used in many training courses. It is effective because it makes a situation seem more realistic. Some people learn well from a book, but most people learn better from experience. Role-playing is a means of giving that experience in a controlled environment. The patient will not feel as though he or she is getting inadequate service. The new optician will not feel the humiliation and/or retaliation from the patient if he or she makes a mistake. In addition, role-playing allows fellow opticians the opportunity to get to know and to help train the new member of the team.

When role-playing, always start with fellow employees acting as the patients. Ask them to come in and act like a typical patient in your store. The new optician should go through the entire process with the "patient," from frame styling and choosing lenses to taking measurements and writing up a bogus job order. Role-play other situations, such as a customer who wants only an adjustment, a patient coming in to pick up her glasses, and even an angry patient with a chip on his shoulder. You need to assess how the optician comes across to patients, as well as his or her ability to perform tasks. During the role-play, you should just observe. Do not make any comments (no matter how tempted you are) until the situation is played out. Then, you need to point out the optician's strong points. After that, tell him or her about areas in which he or she needs improvement. A good way of showing the optician how to improve is to reverse the roles. Have the experienced employee act as the optician and the new optician act as the "patient". Give them a situation to act out. Point out how the experienced person deals with the situation differently. Let the new optician know he or she does not have to repeat word for word what the experienced person says, but he or she should note the difference it made in making a happy situation.

Role-playing is a tool that should be used as much as possible. The most important thing to be learned from role-playing is the interaction between the employee and the patient. Some people have a natural gift for dealing with people and some people need to learn it. Role-playing is sort of a mirror for them to look into and see themselves how other people see them. This is why it is so effective. Knowledge of the products and of the job duties is important, but you need to know how to present it. Role-playing can also be used with current employees to show them a different way of doing things or a more effective way of achieving their goal.

HANDS-ON TRAINING

To teach the optician about frames and frame markings, you should pull several frames off the boards and ask him or her to read the information to you. For example, if the frame is marked 52-18-140; 52 is the eye size, 18 is the bridge size, and 140 is the temple length.

When the optician is learning prescriptions, have him or her read the prescription to you and tell you what each number stands for. For example, if the prescription is –2.00 –0.75 × 159; –2.00 is the sphere (which is the base power), –0.75 is the cylinder (which indicates how much astigmatism the patient has), and 159 is the axis (which is where the cylinder is located).

When the optician is learning to frame style, use a little role-playing and allow him or her to frame style you and other opticians. This will help the new optician (and you) be more confident when he or she is frame styling a patient.

When the optician is learning to take measurements for the lenses, make up several different scenarios of lens styles and frame styles and let him or her practice on you and other opticians. Go through single vision, bifocal, trifocal, and PAL measurements. Allow the optician to master each, one at a time.

To give the optician practice using the lensometer, pull stock lenses and make up several different prescriptions for the optician to "spot". If you have glasses that need to be verified (bifocals, trifocals, and PALs) have the optician check them. This will give him or her practice with the lensometer, as well as practice inspecting the glasses for quality.

ASSESSMENT CHECKLIST

This checklist is to be used after the optician has completed Level 4 in the manual. Observe the optician at work for a week. Mark down his or her level of ability, as well as any comments, in each area. Review the evaluation with the optician once it is complete. Work on weak points together and reinforce strong points.

Task	Needs Work	Qualified	Expert
Answering phones			
Choosing lenses			
Dispensing glasses and contact lenses			
Entering job orders correctly			
Frame styling			
Knowledge of employee benefits			
Knowledge of equipment			
Knowledge of office protocol			
Knowledge of services provided			
Making appointments			
Presentation of lens options			
Presentation of merchandise and services			
Pricing of frames, lenses, contact lenses, examinations, and other services			
Making repairs and adjustments			
Taking measurements			
Troubleshooting			
Use of down time			
Using the lensometer			

Comments:_____

_____

_____

_____

INTERVIEW GUIDELINES FOR THE TRAINER

You should watch for and be aware of the following during the interview:

- Did the prospective employee show up on time? This will give you an idea about whether you can expect him or her to show up on time for work.
- If the prospective employee was late, did he or she call ahead of time to let you know he or she going to be late?
- Is the prospective employee's dress professional or sloppy? This shows you the level of enthusiasm he or she has for working with you.
- How is his or her body language? Nervous? Confident? Bluffer? Anxious? Does not care?

You should start the interview by talking about something unrelated to the job and industry. Getting the prospective employee relaxed enough to talk about himself or herself will let you know more about his or her personality. Some people are nervous during an interview, and you may not be able to see that nervousness. Talk about interests outside of work.

List your expectations of the position you are trying to fill. Tell the prospective employee what your needs are as well as what can be expected from you. Tell the prospective employee the specific job duties expected to be performed and the hours he or she will be expected to work.

Let the new prospect know that there is a future with your company. Tell him or her about the following:

- Future possibilities that may be available
- Benefits your company provides
- Ability to work with employees if a difficult situation arises (e.g., a family emergency).
- Amount the job pays
- Any raises and bonuses that can be expected and how often to expect them

Remember, just as you are interviewing the prospective employee, he or she is interviewing you. He or she does have the option to tell you no and to look elsewhere. If you are up front and honest with the prospective employee about what can be expected from you, you establish trust. That is worth more than money to a lot of people.

Following are some questions to ask the candidate without experience:

- "How did you become interested in optical?"
  You may get a sense of how much he or she knows about optical or what his or her idea is of what you do.
- "What is your past work history?"
  You may get a sense of what types of jobs he or she gravitates toward or what he or she is capable of doing.
- "What do you consider your strengths?"

People like to brag about themselves; listen carefully and you will know if he or she is exaggerating.

- "What do you consider your weaknesses?"
  This will show true character. Be careful though, someone with low self-esteem may exaggerate on this one.
- "How do you best learn information? Reading? Hands-on? A combination of both?"
  You will know how to best teach him or her.
- "In your opinion, what is the most important service an optical store can provide?"
  Again, you will get an idea of what he or she thinks you do.
- "What is the greatest asset you can bring to this team?"
  You will find out how much of a team player he or she may be.
- "What hours are you available to work?"
  You will get a sense of how much he or she is willing to work or situations that may limit the amount of hours he or she can work (e.g., going to school).
- "Tell me a little bit about each place you have worked before. What did you like? What did you not like?"
  You can learn more about his or her attitude and about what you can expect from him or her.

Following are some questions to ask the candidate with experience:

- How did you get started in optical?
- How many years of experience do you have?
- What do you like about it?
- Do you have any certifications? If not, are you interested in becoming certified?
- What are your areas of experience? Optician? Contact lens technician? Ophthalmic technician? Laboratory technician?
- What are your areas of strength?
- What are your areas of weakness?
- Do you have any interest in cross-training? (if he or she has performed only one job duty)
- What equipment have you worked with?
- What assets can you bring to this team?
- What is the average time you spend with a patient?
- What hours are you available to work?
- Tell me a little bit about each place you have worked before. What did you like? What did you not like?

Following are some "test" questions to ask the candidate with experience:

1. Note whether the applicant is wearing an antireflective coating (ARC). If yes, ask "How do you like your ARC?"

If no, ask "Why don't you wear an ARC?"

You will learn two things: (1) Whether he or she knows what ARC stands for. (2) His or her opinion of an ARC.

2. "Do you find it difficult to fit patients with a PAL?"

   If yes, ask him or her to tell you the reasons why.

   If no, ask about his or her method.

   You will learn three things: (1) Whether he or she knows what PAL stands for. (2) Whether he or she needs help in measuring for lenses. (3) Whether he or she has a method that can be shared with the rest of the crew.

3. "How do you handle a difficult patient?" (Give a situation for him or her to handle.)

   You will learn whether you have a follower or a potential leader.

These interview guidelines are just that, a guide. There are probably other specific questions you like to ask. Ask them.

LEVEL 1

New Hire

OBJECTIVES

- Familiarize yourself with your job duties and your employer's expectations of you.
- Learn office procedures and protocol.

> Level 1 may be used for someone with no experience or someone with experience but new to the company.

TASKS TO MASTER

- Introduce yourself to staff members
- Learn office policy and procedures
- Familiarize yourself with time clock
- Learn your **basic job duties**
- Familiarize yourself with **common office equipment**
- Learn **phone protocol**
- Learn the **laboratory process** (if laboratory is on site)
- Learn what the **doctors and doctor's technicians** do (if a doctor is on site)
- Learn prices sheets and how to read them
- Learn how to handle third-party payments, such as those from safety companies, Medicare, and/or insurance

You should have a trainer to follow until you have mastered this level.

LEVEL 1 SCHEDULE

All tasks should be performed as time allows and at the availability of your trainer. A lunch break should be scheduled each day. An assessment should be done at the end of each level to check your progress.

LEVEL 1 NEW HIRE

Stage 1

Task

Become acquainted with fellow staff members and jobs they perform	
Review employee benefits and office protocol	
Learn how to use time clock (manual or computer)	
Read assigned material: *Basic Job Duties*	

Stage 2

Read assigned material: *Common Office Equipment*	
Review price sheets; learn how to read and interrupt them (on examinations, lenses, frame range, contacts, and other services)	

Stage 3

Read assigned material: *Phone Protocol*	
Read assigned material: *Laboratory Process*	

Stage 4

Read assigned material: *Doctors and Technicians*	
Learn how to use the credit card machine(s) and/or postage machine(s)	

Stage 5

Learn how to handle third-party payments (e.g., insurance or safety accounts)	
Complete *Level 1 Assessment* and ask your trainer to review it	

BASIC JOB DUTIES

Job duties vary from location to location, but these are a few of the basic duties of all opticians.

1. Filing charts.
2. Cleaning work area and frame boards.
3. Answering the phone and making appointments.
4. Calling the patient when glasses are ready or when lenses are ready to be cut for the patient's own frame.
5. Following up on jobs for the patient (i.e., checking the status of the job and informing the patient of any delays).
6. Interpreting the prescription. The optician should be able to determine whether the patient needs glasses or contacts.
7. Fitting the patient with lenses that give the best possible vision and have the best fit for his or her lifestyle. This includes tints, anti-reflective coatings (ARCs), safety lenses, progressive lenses, lined bifocals or trifocals, polarized lenses, and thinner lenses.
8. Fitting the patient with the frame that is the best looking, is comfortable, and complements the lenses.
9. Taking measurements from the patient accurately.
10. Consulting and problem solving with patients and other opticians.
11. Adjusting and repairing frames for patients.
12. Dispensing glasses to patients.

> Some opticians (depending on the location) may also do the following:
> Teach patients how to insert and remove contact lenses.
> Instruct patients on wear and care of contact lenses.
> Perform diagnostic tests on patients.

COMMON OFFICE EQUIPMENT

Following is a list of common office equipment you will encounter.

EXAMINATION ROOMS

Topographer   An instrument used to take topographical maps of the front surface of the eye *(cornea)*. It gives the measurements *(curvature and size)* of the cornea and shows the shape *(where and how the curves change)* of the cornea. It is used to map the eye for surgery, it aids in diagnosing some eye diseases, and it can be used to help fit contact lenses.

Auto Refractor   An instrument used to determine the patient's prescription. It reads the curves of the cornea by shooting light at it. The manner in which the light is bounced back determines the prescription. It can also read the cornea for "K" readings *(the curvature of the surface of the cornea)*. It may not be 100% accurate, but it gives the doctor a starting point from which to begin his or her examination.

Auto Keratometer   An instrument that automatically measures the curvatures of the front surface of the eye by shooting light at the cornea and measuring the light that bounces back.

Manual Keratometer   An instrument that manually measures the curvatures of the cornea. As with the lensometer, you have to use power drums and axis wheels and must line up crosshairs when looking at the patient's eye.

Phoropter   An instrument used by the doctor in the examination room to determine the patient's prescription. It looks like a big mask.

Tonopen   A handheld instrument that measures the pressure of the fluid buildup in the eye by tapping the surface of the eye. It is used in testing for glaucoma. This type of test is normally performed on every patient.

Slit Lamp   An instrument used to closely examine the surface of the eye and the back of the eye. It can also be used to take incredibly accurate pressures of the eye in testing for glaucoma.

LABORATORY

Calipers   A tool used to measure the thickness of a lens, either in the center or on the edge.

Lensometer   An instrument that "reads" the prescription (power) of glasses. It looks like a microscope. You have to line up the crosshairs in the center and find the power and axis by using the power drum and axis wheel. Sometimes referred to as a *manual lensometer*.

Edger   An instrument used to cut the lens to the correct shape and size of the frame. Some edgers use patterns for the frame and others trace the frame itself.

Dye Pot   A container used to apply tints to lenses, a process much like that used to dye eggs.

Lens Clock   A handheld instrument used to read the base curve of the lenses.

DISPENSARY

Pupillometer   An instrument used to automatically measure pupillary distances of the patient. It looks similar to a pair of binoculars.

Auto Lensometer   An instrument used to "read" the prescription (power) of the glasses by placing the glasses under a beam of light.

LABORATORY AND DISPENSARY

PD Stick or Ruler   A ruler marked in centimeters and millimeters to manually measure pupillary distances (PD), segment heights for bifocals and trifocals, and frame dimensions.

Screwdriver   A screwdriver made especially for the small screws used in optical frames. It is available in a flat head and a Phillips head.

Flat/Round Nylon Pliers   A tool used to adjust temples of a frame (pull them in and out).

Wide-Jaw Angular Pliers   A tool used to adjust temples of a frame (pull them up and down).

Plastic (Zyle) Shaping Pliers   A tool used to move the temples of a frame up and down. It usually is used on a plastic frame, but it can also be used on a metal frame.

Pad Arm Pliers or Nose Pad Pliers   A tool used to adjust individual nose pads in, out, up, down, forward, and backward.

Nose Pliers or Needle Nose Pliers   A tool that is available in different lengths and thicknesses. It serves many purposes. It can be used to adjust nose pads and temples of frames and to grab screws.

Lens-Aligning Pliers or Lens Turners   A tool used to grip and turn the lens to straighten bifocals or to align the axis when the lens is already mounted in the frame.

Cutting Pliers   A tool used to cut temples of frames, screws, and just about anything else.

PHONE PROTOCOL

Phone protocol is one of the most important skills to be mastered. When a patient calls, you are making his or her first impression of yourself and the office. This is the first encounter the patient has with your office, and it really can make a difference whether that patient decides to come in, make an appointment, or even call back.

It is important that you are perceived professionally while talking to a patient on the phone. The way to do this is to be confident in your answers, happy to be helping, concerned about the caller, and courteous. This makes a good impression not only on the caller but also on the other patients you may have within earshot. Remember, patients are always listening and watching you too. This lets them know how they should expect to be treated. A good rule of thumb is to treat patients how you would like to be treated.

Following is a list of some helpful things you can do while on the phone to ensure you are giving good service:

1. Always have a pen in your hand and paper ready to take down any information necessary. You will usually have something to write down, so by being prepared you will not waste time looking for a piece of paper or a pen. You will appear competent and efficient.
2. Always thank the patient for calling the clinic or office.
3. State the name of the clinic or office.
4. State your name.

> Example of a BASIC SCRIPT: "Thank you for calling ABC Optical, my name is Jane. How may I help you?"

5. Ask "*How* may I help you?" not "*Can* I help you?" Saying the word *can* implies that you may not be able to help—you may not have the knowledge of what to do. However, by saying "HOW may I help you?" you are implying that you DO have the knowledge and are capable of handling whatever the caller may throw at you.
6. Always write down the patient's name. If you did not understand the name when he or she said it, ask "And how do you spell that?" If you ask, "What was that again?" it gives the impression that you are not paying attention. Asking how to spell it shows the caller that you want to get it right. Writing the patient's name down the first time you hear it allows you to repeat it back to the patient without having to ask him or her for it again. This shows a personal interest in the patient and that you are focused on him or her. People like to hear their name, and it makes them feel important. You will establish a "personal" relationship with them and earn their trust. This allows you to offer solutions to their problems without resistance. The patient feels as if you are on his or her side and is happy to be talking to you.
7. When a patient tells you his or her problem, always repeat back the information in your own words. This allows you to be sure you

understand exactly what the problem is, and the patient feels that you understand his or her situation.

8. If finding a solution to the problem is going to take longer than 30 seconds, take down a phone number where you can reach the patient with the correct information or solution. Explain to the patient that it may take a while and you would rather not put him or her on hold the whole time. This shows that you are being considerate of the patient's time and feelings. Some people are calling from their mobile phone and would rather stay on hold. That is all right if you have explained to the caller that there will be a wait.

9. Above all, *smile, smile, smile*. Smiling the whole time you are on the phone makes it sound as if you are happy even if you are not.

> Keep in mind the entire time you are on the phone, any and all other patients in the store are listening to and watching you. They get a sense of how they can expect to be treated by the way you treat the patient on the phone.

LABORATORY PROCESS

The two main parts of an optical laboratory are surfacing and finishing. A *surfacing laboratory* is where the lenses are actually made by molding, casting, or grinding the prescription into the lens. They are made to order. When the lens is completed here, it has the prescription in it but is just one large "blank." In the *finishing laboratory*, the lenses are cut down from the blanks to fit the size and shape of the frame and are placed at the measurements you took from the patient.

IN THE SURFACING LABORATORY

1. The lens starts as a semifinished blank, meaning the prescription has not been ground in yet. The necessary blank is chosen for the type of lens (e.g., bifocal, single vision) and the appropriate base curve is chosen. Lens blanks come in different sizes: 70, 75, and 80 mm.

2. The base curve, the measurements of the frame, the patient's measurements, and the prescription are input into the computer.

3. The back curve cuts, tools, and thickness are then calculated.

4. The lens is appropriately marked and blocked.

5. The generators are set to the correct curves for the front and back curves, the tools are put in place, and the desired thickness is set.

6. The lens is then cut to the correct prescription. This process is done slowly so as not to put waves, scratches, or cracks into the lens.
7. Next the lens is polished: It goes through three finishing stages to ensure that it is polished to transparency and that no waves or scratches are on the lens.
8. The lens is then cleaned and inspected to ensure that the prescription and base curve are correct and that there are no defects.
9. From here, it is sent to the finishing laboratory.

> All ARCs and some tints are added to the lens in the surfacing laboratory before it reaches the finishing laboratory.

IN THE FINISHING LABORATORY

1. The lens is again inspected so that the optical centers can be located *(spotted)* and the prescription verified. The lens is also checked for scratches, defects, and prismatic effect. ARCs and/or tints are applied, if specified for that particular job, and are verified at this time.
2. Next the calculations are done to ensure that placement of the lens in the frame matches the measurements taken from the patient (e.g., PD, segment height, ocular height).
3. The lens is then laid out and "blocked up". This means that a metal chuck is adhered to the lens. This metal chuck allows the lens to be placed in the edger for the cutting process.
4. Once the lens is blocked, it is cut to the shape and size of the frame. On some edgers you have to pull a pattern for the frame and on others the frame is traced. The appropriate bevel is also cut (metal, plastic, rimless, or drill mount).
5. If the lens needs to be grooved or drilled to mount in the frame, that is done after the size and shape are cut.
6. After the lens is cut any coatings that are needed (e.g., tints, ultraviolet [UV] and hard coatings) are applied. Before an ARC is applied, if the job calls for it, the tints and/or UV coatings should have been applied and verified already.
7. Next the lenses are mounted into the frame and inspected again to make sure all of the measurements are correct and no scratches or defects are present.

The preceding section presented a brief overview of what is done in a laboratory. The basic process may take longer depending on the type of equipment your laboratory uses. Going through a laboratory to see this process helps you appreciate all that goes into making a pair of glasses. If you have the opportunity to watch the process, it is highly recommended that you do so. It will help you better understand what goes into making a pair of glasses and how to work for your patients.

DOCTORS AND TECHNICIANS

If you have a doctor in your office, it would benefit you greatly to talk with him or her and to follow him or her, as well as the technicians, through their process.

DOCTOR

The doctor is the beginning and end of all treatments for the patient.
Following is a list of the doctor's common duties.

1. Refracts (i.e., determines the patient's prescription for glasses and/or contact lenses)
2. Tests for all eye diseases, conditions, and/or disorders
3. Administers medications when needed for eye conditions and/or diseases
4. Administers any necessary treatments for eye conditions and/or diseases
5. Fits patients for contact lenses
6. Provides postoperative care (e.g., for cataract surgery, refractive surgery) to patients of some surgeons

TECHNICIAN

The technician is basically the doctor's assistant.
Following is a list of the technician's common duties.

1. Takes the history of the patient and determines his or her chief complaint.
2. Runs diagnostic tests and takes acuities.
3. Administers drops as directed by the doctor.
4. Teaches patients how to insert and remove contact lenses.
5. Teaches patients how to wear and care for their contact lenses.
6. Keeps the flow of patients going for the doctor.

Every person is important in the process of helping the patient obtain the best possible glasses and vision. The staff is involved in the process in the following order:

1. Technician
2. Doctor
3. Dispenser
4. Laboratory technician
5. Back to dispenser

You can see we all play our part. We are all important. We work together as a team.

LEVEL 1 ASSESSMENT

1. True or False: One of your basic job duties is to dispense glasses.
2. At some locations, the optician will:
   A. Figure payroll
   B. Teach patients how to insert and remove contact lenses
   C. Clean the Phoropter
   D. Do paperwork at the end of the day
3. Although some job duties vary from location to location, most opticians will:
   A. Do maintenance work on all of the equipment
   B. Check the patient for eye diseases
   C. Determine the patient's prescription
   D. Fit the patient with frames and lenses
4. True or False: Doing adjustments are a part of everyday duties for an optician.
5. A lensometer measures:
   A. The front curvature of the lens
   B. The prescription of the lens
   C. The surface of the cornea
   D. The distance between the pupils
6. A lens turner (or lens-aligning pliers) is found in the:
   A. Laboratory
   B. Examination room
   C. Dispensary
   D. Laboratory and dispensary
7. A Phoropter is an instrument that is used by the:
   A. Doctor
   B. Laboratory technician
   C. Dispenser
   D. Receptionist
8. What instrument is used to measure the distance between the pupils?
   A. Slit lamp
   B. Caliper
   C. Pupillometer
   D. Keratometer
9. What should you always have when answering the phone?
   A. Tools
   B. The patient chart
   C. Pen and paper
   D. Job orders and payment
10. True or False: You make your first impression on patients when they come in to pick up their glasses.

11. When talking to a patient on the phone, a good rule of thumb is to:
    A. Tell the patient you are busy and you will call him or her back later
    B. Treat the patient like you would want to be treated
    C. Put the patient on hold for as long as it takes
    D. Ask the patient "Can I help you?"
12. When the patient states his or her problem:
    A. Tell him or her to hold
    B. Repeat it back to him or her to clarify
    C. Refer him or her to someone else
    D. Make an appointment for a contact lens examination
13. What are the two main parts of an optical laboratory?
14. In the surfacing laboratory:
    A. The lens is cut to the size and shape of the frame
    B. The prescription is ground into the lens
    C. The groove is put into the lens
    D. The frame color is determined
15. In the finishing laboratory:
    A. The prescription is ground into the lens
    B. All ARCs are applied
    C. The lenses are polished on the back side
    D. The lenses are cut to the correct size and shape of the frame
16. True or False: The frame is picked out once it is sent off to the laboratory.
17. True or False: The technicians perform diagnostic testing for the doctors.
18. The doctor will:
    A. Test for eye diseases
    B. Determine the patient's prescription
    C. Treat eye diseases and conditions
    D. All of the above
19. When a patient calls the office, which person makes the first impression?
    A. Laboratory technician
    B. Doctor's technician
    C. Doctor
    D. Optician
20. True or False: The doctor's job and the dispensing optician's job never affect one another

LEVEL 2

Office Assistant (Working with Patients)

OBJECTIVES

- Begin your education on becoming an optician.
- Learn how to handle questions from patients in person and on the phone.
- Learn how to ensure a good patient flow and how to provide good service.

TASKS TO MASTER

- Begin answering phones and **making appointments**
- Learn about and practice quoting prices
- Familiarize yourself with the frame lines carried in your office
- Learn about **the eye**
- Learn about **eye conditions**
- Learn about **light and refraction**
- Learn about different **frames**
- Learn how to make **adjustments**
- Learn about **lenses**
- Learn about **lens coatings and extras**
- Learn about contact lenses

All of your work should be double-checked and your education should be monitored until you have mastered this level.

LEVEL 2 SCHEDULE

In Level 2, the tasks are to be done with close supervision. An assessment should be given to check your progress.

LEVEL 2 OFFICE ASSISTANT (WORKING WITH PATIENTS)

Task

Stage 1

Read assigned material: *Making Appointments*	
Begin answering phones and making appointments	
Practice quoting prices	
Familiarize yourself with frame lines carried in your office	

Stage 2

Continue answering phones and making appointments	
Read assigned material: *The Eye*	
Read assigned material: *Eye Conditions*	
Read assigned material: *Light and Refraction*	

Stage 3

Continue answering phones and making appointments	
Read assigned material: *Frames*	
Read assigned material: *Adjustments*	
Start doing adjustments on patients' frames	

Stage 4

Continue answering phones and making appointments	
Continue doing adjustments on patients' frames	
Read assigned material: *Lenses*	
Read assigned material: *Lens Coatings and Extras*	

Stage 5

Continue answering phones and making appointments	
Continue doing adjustments on patients' frames	
Read assigned material: *Contact Lenses*	
Complete *Level 2 Assessment* and ask your trainer to review it	

MAKING APPOINTMENTS

When a patient calls and wants to make an appointment, use the phone protocol that you learned in Level 1.

Following is a guideline to use when making appointments.

1. Ask the patient whether he or she needs an appointment for an annual eye examination for glasses or contact lenses. If the patient needs to see the doctor because of a specific problem, he or she usually volunteers this information at this time. If not, you may inquire as to the reason for the appointment. For example, the patient's eyes may be itchy or watering a lot and he or she may want to see the doctor. Some patients have an eye injury. In the case of an actual injury to the eye, it usually is best for the patient to go to the emergency room to get patched before he or she goes to the optometrist. It depends on the severity of the injury.

2. Ask the patient whether he or she prefers a morning or an afternoon appointment.

3. If there is more than one doctor in your office, ask the patient whether he or she has a preference about which doctor he or she sees. *(He or she may be a long-term patient of a particular doctor and wish to continue with that doctor.)* At this time, you will state the next available appointment with that doctor. It is important that you say, "My next available appointment with Dr. Smith is Wednesday, May 15 at 2:00." Do not tell a patient that the doctor is not in or is on vacation. The patient is not interested in that. He or she wants to know the earliest possible time he or she can get an appointment with the doctor of his or her choice. It also makes your office sound more professional. It is also important that you state the *day, date,* and *time* of the appointment when you are scheduling.

4. If the patient has never been to your office, tell him or her your next available appointment and the doctor's name (e.g., "My next available appointment is Wednesday, May 15 at 2:00 with Dr. Smith."). You should also get the patient's *full name, address, phone number,* and *date of birth.* This way you can start the appropriate paperwork before the patient arrives for his or her appointment.

5. At the end of the conversation, after the appointment has been made, repeat back to the patient the day, date, and time of the appointment. Thank the patient for calling and using your store. Tell him or her that you will call the day before the appointment to confirm it.

Your office may already have someone designated for making appointments. Check with your trainer to see whether this will be one of your responsibilities.

THE EYE

This section presents some of the major parts of the eye with which you need to be familiar. However, the eye is much more complex; this chapter covers only the basics.

Cornea The clear membrane over the iris and limbus. It is responsible for most of the refraction *(bending)* of light in the eye. It is approximately 0.8 mm thick and consists of the following five layers.

Epithethium The outermost layer of the cornea; it renews itself repeatedly.

Bowman's Membrane Membrane found directly beneath the epithelium; it holds in the next layer.

Stroma The thickest part of the cornea; it is found directly under Bowman's membrane.

Descemet's Membrane Membrane found directly under the stroma; it holds in the other side of the stroma.

Endothelium The innermost layer of the cornea; it prevents the fluid behind the retina from getting into the cornea.

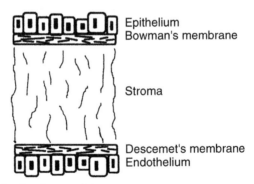

FIGURE 2-1 The five layers of the cornea.

Eyelid The flap of skin that covers the eye when you blink, close your eyes, or are asleep.

Iris The colored part of the eye.

Limbus   The black ring around the iris.

Pupil   The opening in the middle of the eye through which light passes.

Sclera   The white part of the eye. It is composed of a fibrous tissue that helps maintain the shape of the eye.

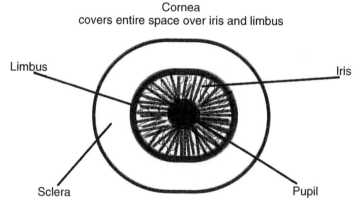

FIGURE 2-2 The eye (outside, front view).

Aqueous Humor   The watery fluid found behind the cornea and in front of the iris. This chamber is known as the *anterior chamber.*

Choroid   Located between the sclera and the retina, this part of the eye is full of veins and provides oxygen and nutrients through blood flow to the retina and the sclera.

Ciliary Body   A part of the eye that is connected to and is located in front of the choroid. Included in the ciliary body are the ciliary processes, which are responsible for making the aqueous fluid that fills the chamber in front of the iris and behind the cornea.

Lens   Located inside the eye behind the pupil, this part of the eye helps with the refraction *(bending)* of light passing through the eye.

Optic Nerve   Nerve that sends the information from the retina to the back of the brain and tells you what you are seeing.

Retina   Located in the innermost layer of the eye, the retina is where the picture is made of what the eye is seeing.

Vitreous Fluid   The jellylike fluid that fills the inside of the eyeball and gives the eyeball its shape.

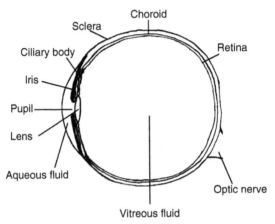

Figure 2-3 The eye (side view).

The retina is composed of many parts that create the images we see.

Cones   Photoreceptors that handle color vision and sharpness of images. They are stimulated by brighter lighting conditions. Most of them are located in the macula and fovea.

Rods   Photoreceptors that handle vision in dim lighting or during "night" vision; they do not distinguish colors as the cones do. They are sensitive to motion and most of them are located in the peripheral *(outer)* sides of the retina.

Macula   Located in the central part of the retina, it is made up of the highest concentration of rods and cones.

Fovea   A small area in the middle of the macula where there are no rods. Because cones handle sharpness of images, this area allows you to see the detail in the image.

Optic Disc   Located to the side of the macula, this disc contains no rods and cones. It commonly is referred to as the *blind spot.*

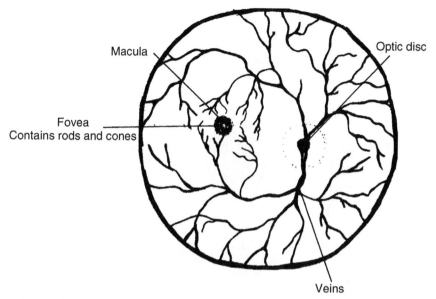

FIGURE 2-4 The eye (inside back view of retina).

There are six major muscles surrounding the eye, which move the globe in several different directions. Using combinations of these muscles, the eye can move in almost any direction. The following definitions are given to help you remember some of their names and locations.

Superior Rectus   Muscle that moves the eye up and in. It is attached on the top of the eye globe.

Inferior Rectus   Muscle that moves the eye down and in. It is attached on the bottom of the eye globe.

External Rectus   Muscle that moves the eye out toward the temple. It is attached on the outside *(temporal side)* of the eye globe.

Internal Rectus   Muscle that moves the eye in toward the nose. It is attached on the inside *(nasal side)* of the eye globe.

Superior Oblique   Muscle that moves the eye down and out. It is attached between the superior rectus and the internal rectus.

Inferior Oblique   Muscle that moves the eye up and out. It is attached between the internal rectus and the inferior rectus.

Superior   Usually means to be on the top.

Inferior   Usually means to be on the bottom.

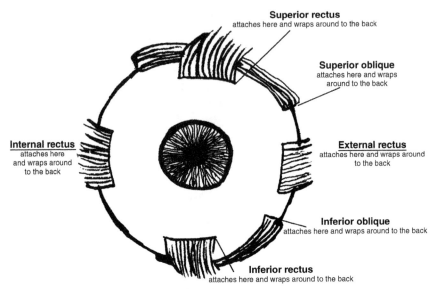

Superior rectus
attaches here and wraps around to the back

Superior oblique
attaches here and wraps
around to the back

Internal rectus
attaches here
and wraps around
to the back

External rectus
attaches here and wraps around
to the back

Inferior oblique
attaches here and wraps around to the back

Inferior rectus
attaches here and wraps around to the back

FIGURE 2-5 The eye muscles (left eye).

EYE CONDITIONS

An eye condition is a circumstance in which the eye has developed poorly, usually resulting in poor vision or discomfort. Conditions of the eye are usually treatable with either corrective lenses or medication. Following is a list of a few of the more common eye conditions.

Ametropia A term meaning that the patient needs some type of visual correction with prescription lenses.

Amblyopia A condition in which the eye is not able to function normally. Rather than straining, the eye does what is called *suppressing the image*. The affected eye accommodates itself to receive the best possible image and the other eye ignores the image. Even with the best possible corrective lenses, the patient's vision still will not be 20/20. This normally occurs only in one eye.

Anisometropia A condition in which the patient requires unequal amounts of correction from one eye to the other (e.g., one eye may be a plus prescription and the other a minus prescription, or the difference in the amount of correction needed from one eye to the next is more than 2 to 3 diopters).

Astigmatism A condition in which one of two things has happened: Either the cornea has two different curves rather than a singular curve over the entire surface, or the eyeball is shaped like a football. The result is, the patient sees two different images. Therefore he or she requires a cylindrical lens (e.g., −1.00 −0.50 × 89 instead of −1.00 sphere only).

There are five different types of astigmatism.

Simple Myopic Astigmatism   A condition in which one image falls on the retina and the other image falls in front of the retina.

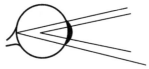

Figure 2-6 Simple myopic astigmatism.

Simple Hyperopic Astigmatism   A condition in which one image falls on the retina and the other image falls behind the retina.

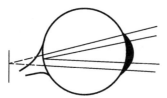

Figure 2-7 Simple hyperopic astigmatism.

Compound Myopic Astigmatism   A condition in which both images fall in front of the retina in two different spots.

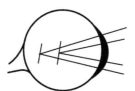

Figure 2-8 Compound myopic astigmatism.

Compound Hyperopic Astigmatism   A condition in which both images fall behind the retina in two different spots.

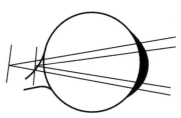

Figure 2-9 Compound hyperopic astigmatism.

Mixed Astigmatism A condition in which one image falls in front of the retina and the other image falls behind the retina.

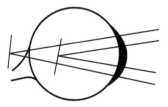

FIGURE 2-10 Mixed astigmatism.

Aphakia A condition resulting from a person having surgery for cataracts, in which a new, man-made lens was never put in to take the place of the old one. Patients with aphakia wear a lenticular lens to compensate for the refractive power the natural lens inside the eye provided. The lens looks like it has a bubble in the middle and flat plastic around the edge. The power of these lenses is usually approximately +13.00 to +19.00.

Binocular Vision A condition in which the two eyes are taking the images and putting them together to make one image (i.e., both eyes work together to see the same image in the brain).

Cataract A condition in which the natural lens inside the eye has become so clouded *(opaque)* and hardened that vision is impaired greatly. Unless surgery is performed to correct this, glasses will no longer help the patient's vision become clear.

Diplopia A condition in which the patient has double vision, or sees the same image but in two different places at the same time. The eyes are not working together to produce one solid image. In this case the eyes are using *monocular* vision. The eyes are working separately and not together as with *binocular* vision.

Emmetropia The state in which the eye is completely normal and does *not* require any correction with lenses.

Esophoria A condition in which one or both of the eyes have the tendency to turn in toward the nose in comparison with each other. The eye occasionally turns in toward the nose; it does not stay that way all the time.

Esotropia A condition in which one or both of the eyes turn in toward the nose. The doctor usually prescribes a lens with prism or visual therapy to correct this problem. The eyes usually stay turned in all the time.

Exophoria A condition in which one or both of the eyes have the tendency to turn out toward the ears in comparison with each other. The eye occasionally turns out toward the ear; it does not stay that way all the time.

Exotropia A condition in which one or both of the eyes turn out toward the ears. The doctor usually prescribes a lens with prism or visual therapy to correct this problem. The eyes usually stay turned out all the time. Use the following tools to remember the differences between *-tropia* and *-phoria.*

-tropia: The condition is usually permanent. It can be corrected with treatment. Think "trapped."

-phoria: The condition is temporary. The condition will occur but not remain fixed. Treatment is not always necessary. Think "fear" or "phobia."

Glaucoma A condition in which the pressure of the fluid in the anterior chamber of the eye builds up because the channels are blocked and the fluid is not allowed to be released. The result is possible vision loss. Glaucoma is usually treatable with medication.

Hyperopia The condition of being farsighted (i.e., the image the eye receives falls behind the retina, and the patient can clearly see objects that are far away but not those that are near). The patient wears plus lenses for correction.

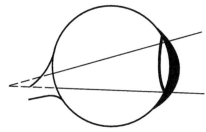

FIGURE 2-11 Hyperopia.

Myopia The condition of being nearsighted (i.e., the image the eye receives falls in front of the retina, and the patient can clearly see objects that are close up but not those that are far away). The patient wears minus lenses for correction.

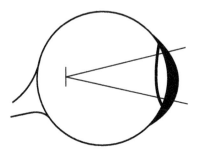

FIGURE 2-12 Myopia.

Photophobia   The condition of being abnormally sensitive to light, both indoors and outdoors.

Presbyopia   The loss of the eye's ability to accommodate for close-up work or reading. The patient has to wear bifocals for correction. This condition usually affects everyone after the age of 40.

Strabismus   The condition of one or both eyes not being in correct alignment when at rest. This is usually because the muscles controlling the movement of the eye are not working correctly. This results in the patient seeing two different images *(diplopia)*. If this condition is not corrected early enough, it could result in *amblyopia* (suppressing the image in one eye, so vision is impaired). Strabismus is usually corrected with prism in corrective lenses and/or vision therapy.

LIGHT AND REFRACTION

LIGHT

There are several theories on how light travels. We follow and use the *Electromagnetic Light Theory*. This theory states that light travels in *waves* away from the light source to the object.

All light travels at the same speed, which is 186,000 miles/sec. Each wave of light has a different *wavelength*. Wavelength is the distance from the top of one wave to the top of the next wave; it is measured in *nanometers*. A nanometer is one one-billionth of a meter. There are many different wavelengths; some we see and some we do not see. The wavelengths that you do see are colors. The wavelengths you do not see are ultraviolet (UV) and infrared light. The difference between UV and infrared light and colors is the distance between the wavelengths. If the wavelength is shorter, the light is less visible. If the wavelength is longer, the light is more visible.

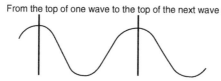

FIGURE 2-13 Wavelength.

NONVISIBLE LIGHT

There are three types of UV light. Their wavelengths, which range between 200 and 400 nm, are shorter than the wavelengths of colors. Any light with a wavelength lower than 200 nm is usually absorbed and/or filtered out by the cornea.

UVA	200-275 nm
UVB	275-300 nm
UVC	300-400 nm

UV light between 300 and 400 nm is usually absorbed by the crystalline lens inside the eye. The lens naturally hardens and becomes opaque as we get older. This process can actually speed up if the patient has been exposed to excessive UV light. This is why you should always recommend that your patients get UV filters on their lenses.

VISIBLE LIGHT

Colors have longer wavelengths than UV light. The wavelengths of colors range between approximately 400 and 750 nm. Violet has the shortest wavelength and red has the longest.

Violet	400-465 nm
Blue	460-500 nm
Green	501-560 nm
Yellow	561-590 nm
Orange	591-650 nm
Red	651-750 nm

A wavelength higher than 751 nm is considered infrared light. It is better known as *heat energy*.

As stated previously, light travels at 186,000 miles/sec in air. Any time light enters a new medium, such as water, plastic, or glass, it slows and bends. The bending of light is called *refraction*. The only time the light is not bent is when the light hits the new medium straight ahead at a perpendicular angle (exactly 90 degrees away from the surface of the medium).

Three things affect how much light is bent:

1. The *thickness* of the medium
2. The *density* (how close together the molecules are) of the medium
3. The *angle* at which light hits the medium. Some light is bent going through the medium, but some light can hit the surface at such an angle that it is *reflected* (bounced back off the lens).

The density of optical lenses is also referred to as the *refractive index*. You can find charts that list the refractive index for most materials used in making glasses. Many of these charts vary because the speed of light in a given material may change because of the makeup of that material. However, you should find that the numbers on different charts are almost the same (e.g., the refractive index for plastic may be listed as 1.52 on one chart and as 1.50 on another chart). Following is an easy formula to use to figure the refractive index:

Refractive index = Speed of light in air ÷ Speed of light in material

Index 1.53 = 186,000 miles/sec ÷ 121,569 miles/sec

You will not have to calculate the refractive index often. However, you will often hear the index of refraction being referred to when you deal with the "thinner and lighter" lenses that are available (e.g., polycarbonate). The higher the refractive index, the thinner the lens will be. Technology is changing constantly, and manufacturers introduce thinner lenses all the time. The thinnest polycarbonate lens or high index lens that used to be available had a 1.60 refractive index, now there is a lens with a 1.66 index that is available.

Following are the four basic materials used in making glasses, along with their index of refraction:

Plastic	1.52
Glass	1.56
High index	1.60-1.66
Polycarbonate	1.60-1.66

There are many more types or variations of these materials, because all manufacturers produce their own versions.

REFRACTION

An ophthalmic lens is designed as if two prism wedges were put together, with each prism wedge having a *base* and an *apex*.

Prism   A wedge of transparent material (plastic or glass) that bends light.

Base   The thickest part of the wedge. Light bends toward the base of a lens. The viewed image moves away from the base when the lens is moved.

Apex The thinnest part of the wedge. Light bends away from the apex of a lens. The viewed image moves toward the apex when the lens is moved.

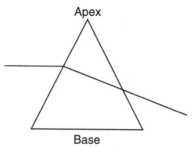

FIGURE 2-14 Prism wedge.

The thicker the lens, the more light is bent. The denser the lens, the more light is bent. Both of these result in a stronger powered lens. The opposite also holds true. The thinner the lens, the less light is bent. The less dense the material, the less light is bent. Both of these result in a weaker powered lens.

Diopter The unit of measure used to express the power of the lens (e.g., –2.00 is the same as minus two diopters).

Lenses have a minimum of two curves, which also affect the refraction of the light before it reaches the eye. There is the front surface curve (also known as the *base curve*) and the back surface curve. The front surface curvature is convex and there is usually only one solid curve over the entire front surface of the lens. The back surface curvature is concave and can be one solid curve like the front, or it may have two curves.

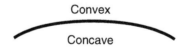

FIGURE 2-15 Lens curve.

There are three different types of lens curve designs: spherical, cylindrical, and aspheric. Each one tells you what type of prescription or what type of condition a patient may have. You will learn more about these three types in the section about base curves.

Vertex Distance The distance between the back surface of the lens and the front surface of the eye.

Vertex distance

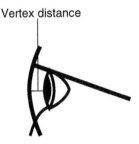

FIGURE 2-16 Vertex distance.

The vertex distance is important to the doctor when he or she is in the examination room figuring the prescription for the patient. Because of the properties of lenses, the power of the lenses is greatly affected the closer or farther away they sit from the eyes. The power of the lens may become stronger or weaker depending on the prescription and distance. This is the reason a patient's contact lens prescription is usually different from his or her glasses prescription. The contact lens sits directly on the eye and the glasses sit away from the eye.

In summary, four major factors determine the overall power of a lens and how well the lens bends light.

1. Thickness
2. Density
3. Curvature (front and back)
4. Distance

To learn more detail about light and refraction, please read the textbooks *Professional Dispensing for Opticianry* (Opticians Association of America Staff, 1996) and *Understanding Lens Surfacing* (CW Brooks, 1992), both available from Elsevier.

FRAMES

A measurement   The horizontal measurement of the frame from the farthest inside nasal point to the farthest inside temporal point of the frame. This is usually called the *eye size* of the frame *(width)*.

B measurement   The vertical measurement of the frame from the farthest inside top point of the frame to the farthest inside bottom point of the frame *(depth)*.

ED measurement   The diagonal measurement of the frame. The most common method of taking this measurement is to take the longest diagonal measurement from the farthest inside nasal point of the frame down to the farthest inside temporal point of the frame. The more accurate and more technical definition is twice the longest radius measuring from the geometric center of the frame to the farthest point inside the frame.

DBL (Distance Between Lenses). The measurement from the inside nasal point of one "eye" to the inside nasal point of the other "eye." DBL is also known as the *bridge size*.

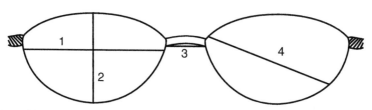

1. A Measurement - Eye size
2. B Measurement - up and down
3. DBL Measurement - Bridge size
4. ED Measurement - diagonal

FIGURE 2-17 Frame measurements. **1**, A measurement (eye size). **2**, B measurement (up and down). **3**, DBL measurement (bridge size). **4**, ED measurement (diagonal).

Measurements of a frame will always be taken from an inside point to another inside point of the frame. When taking measurements of a frame, you never include the measurement of the frame itself because each frame varies in thickness. This can lead to inaccuracy in lens placement, thickness, and segment heights.

Temple The long side piece of the frame that hooks around the ear. Sometimes it is referred to as the *arm*. There are three basic types:

Skull or standard   Bends with ear
Cable   Wraps around the ear
Library or paddle   Goes straight back; stays close to the head

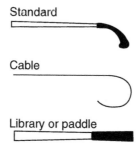

Standard

Cable

Library or paddle

FIGURE 2-18 Temple styles.

Temple Length   The length of the temple in millimeters: 130, 135, 140, 145, 150, 155, and rarely, 160 (160 is usually found only in cable temples). Each manufacturer usually has three or four lengths available for each frame style.

Temple Tip   The plastic end piece on the temple to protect the ear.

Spring Hinges   The type of hinges found in some frames. The springs in the temple allow the frame to bounce back and stretch out farther if bumped, or allow better fit for comfort.

Eye Wire   The metal or plastic part of the frame that goes around the lenses.

Bridge   The piece in the middle of the frame that connects the two eye pieces (DBL).

Nose Pads   Pads that rest directly on the nose for support. There are three basic types of nose pads, and most of them adjust to the nose.

Mount   To put lenses in frames.

Dismount   To take lenses out of frames.

Face Form   The shape of the front of the frame; it is made to fit the contour of the patient's face. If you look down on a patient from the top, it should "wrap" around the face a little. Hence, it is also called *facial wrap*.

Top view of patient's head

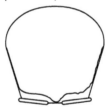

Face form (facial wrap)

FIGURE 2-19 Face form.

Shifted   Either the nose pads or the temples are going to the left or the right instead of being evenly spread out.

Pantoscopic Tilt   When a patient is viewed from the side, the frame is at an angle such that the bottom of the frame is closer to the face than the top. This is the most common fit for a frame.

Retroscopic Tilt   When a patient is viewed from the side, the frame is at an angle such that the top of the frame is closer to the face than the bottom.

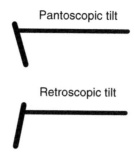

Pantoscopic tilt

Retroscopic tilt

FIGURE 2-20 Frame tilt.

TYPES OF FRAMES

Metal   Frame made of metal alloy (a combination of different types of metals); referred to as a *full frame*, meaning that the frame goes all the way around the lens.

Plastic   Frame made of plastic (also called a *Zyle frame*); referred to as a *full frame*, meaning that the frame goes all the way around the lens. You may heat the frame to manipulate the shape and/or size to put the lens in or take the lens out of the frame.

Optyl   Frame made of a type of plastic that *cannot* be heated because heat warps the shape of the frame or melts the frame completely. It is also a full frame.

Titanium   Metal frame made of titanium. This frame is more flexible and durable than an ordinary metal frame. In addition, it is good for patients who have an allergic reaction to regular metal frames that contain nickel. Titanium frames are known for being lightweight.

Stainless Steel   Metal frame made of stainless steel, which is more flexible and durable than regular metal but not as tough as titanium. In addition, it is good for patients who have an allergic reaction to regular metal frames.

Rimless   Frame that has metal surrounding the lens on the top half and wire on the bottom half. The lens has to be grooved and a "fishing wire" is used to hold the lens in at the bottom of the frame. The lens is exposed on the bottom half. It is also called *semirimless*.

Drill Mount   Frame that comes in pieces, usually two temples and a nosepiece. The lenses have holes drilled into them to attach the frame pieces. There are two basic types of drill mounts: four hole and three piece.

Safety   Frames that are made according to OSHA standards. They are made for people who work in factories or in other environments that demand the eyes be protected. Titmus and Hudson are common manufacturers of safety frames.

The aforementioned types of frames are available in many variations. Only the basic types have been presented.

TYPES OF NOSEPIECES

Individual Pads   Metal pieces welded onto the frame. The nose pads either screw onto or snap into the metal piece. They are the most adjustable to the patient's nose and bridge.

Saddle Bridge   One solid piece that connects from one side of the frame to the other and either screws or snaps on.

Soft Wing   Piece much like the saddle bridge, except it is adjustable to the bridge of the nose. There are metal pieces inside the silicone pad, which allows it to be adjusted.

TYPES OF NOSE PADS

There are three different types of nose pads: hard, soft, and silicon. There are two different shapes of nose pads: -shaped (shaped like a to fit right and left) and symmetrical (oval shaped to fit either right or left).

HOW TO READ INFORMATION ON THE FRAME AND WHERE TO FIND IT

Following is an example of what is written on the temple:

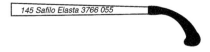

145 Safilo Elasta 3766 055

FIGURE 2-21 Temple reading.

Temple length	145
Manufacturer	Safilo
Frame line and number or name	Elasta 3766
Frame color (may be written in numeric form or letter abbreviation for the color)	055

Following is an example of what is written on the bridge:

59 - 17

FIGURE 2-22 Bridge reading.

Eye size or A measurement	59
Bridge size or DBL	17

The B measurement and the ED measurement must be taken manually with a PD ruler.

Frames are available in six basic shapes:

Oval
Round
Square
Octagon
Aviator
Cat eye

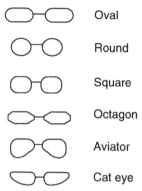

Oval

Round

Square

Octagon

Aviator

Cat eye

FIGURE 2-23 Frame shapes.

> When frame-styling a patient, try to choose a shape opposite the patient's face to make his or her features more balanced.

STANDARD ALIGNMENT OF A FRAME

The standard alignment of a frame is also called the *truing* the frame. This gives you a starting point to go from when adjusting or repairing glasses for a patient.

1. *Temple tips*—your thumb should contour when placed on the underside of the temple tip.
2. *Temples*—should go straight back from the frame front.
3. *Frame front*—should follow the contour of the patient's face; it should not be flat or so curved that it looks like it might break. It should also be level and straight when the frame is turned upside down and laid on the temples. Usually, one temple does not touch the table. To fix this, bend the temples up or down until both of them touch the table.
4. *Nose pads or bridge*—should align with the curve of the frame front, if the frame is metal. In other words, the nose pads should be hidden by the metal of the frame and should not stick out too much when the frame is viewed straight on.

Each patient has a special way he or she likes his or her glasses to fit. The information given here is only a starting point; it is to be used as a basic guideline.

ADJUSTMENTS

Some common complaints are presented in this section; however, the more experience you have, the more you will run into different situations. This section gives you a foundation to handle most situations.

Complaint   "My nose pads hurt and make dents in my nose."
Problem   The nose pads are too close together.
Solution   Spread the nose pads apart a little.

Complaint   "My glasses are always slipping down my nose."
Problem   The glasses are too loose.
Solution   Pull in the temples a little. Bend the temple tips down a little. Pull in the nose pads a little. All of this will make the frame snug to the head. It is better to do a little bending at a time so that you do not end up making the glasses too tight and pinching the patient's head.

Complaint   "I see ghosts [and/or reflections] on the side when I turn my head."
Problem   The lenses are bending away from the face instead of contouring to the face causing the patient to see reflections on the backside of the lens.
Solution   Give the frame more facial wrap and spread the temples slightly so that they do not pinch the patient's head when you wrap the frame.

Complaint   "One lens feels closer to my face than the other one does. One lens touches my cheek."
Problem   The temples are shifted.
Solution   Straighten the temples so that they are going straight back and not leaning to the left or the right.

Complaint   "My glasses touch my cheeks, especially when I smile."
Problem   There is too much pantoscopic tilt in the frame.
Solution   Bend the temples up. This pulls the bottom of the frame away from the cheeks so the frame will not rest on them.

Complaint   "When I blink, my lashes rub against the lenses."
Problem   The lenses are too close to the patient's face.
Solution   Pull in the nose pads a little. Pull the nose pads out away from the frame. Bend the temples down a little. Give the frame a little facial wrap because you are pulling the lenses away from the face and the patient will notice the lenses more.

Complaint   "I can see the line of my bifocal. I always have to drop my head if I want to look out."
Problem   The frame is sitting too high.

Solution   Increase the facial wrap and bend the temples up. Spread out the nose pads. This drops the segment line down approximately 1 to 2 mm. If it looks to be 3 mm or more, you may have to measure again and make new lenses.

When adjusting frames, a good rule of thumb is to imagine how the frame should look, and adjust the frame accordingly. Remember, the patient may want or need the frame to be out of "normal" alignment to compensate for some of his or her unique features.

BASIC WRITTEN EYEGLASS PRESCRIPTION

	Sphere	Cylinder	Axis	Prism
Name: *Lily Smith* Date: *11-15-01*				
Address:				
OD	−3.25	−0.50	145	1.5 BD
OS	−4.25	−1.50	89	2.0 BU
Add	2.00	Comments: *Varilux Comfort w/ ARC*		
Dr. *Mike Jeckle OD*				
Exp. *11-15-02*				

FIGURE 2-24 Basic written eyeglass prescription. *Add*, Additional power for the near correction (if needed); *axis*, location of the cylinder power; *cylinder*, correction for astigmatism (if needed); *OD*, right eye; *OS*, left eye; *prism*, amount of prism needed (if needed); *sphere*, base power of the lens. Read about prisms in the section, More About Lenses, p. 69.

An expiration date should always be written on the prescription. If there is not a date, always check with the prescribing doctor if you have any questions or doubts about the prescription.

LENSES

There are plus lenses and minus lenses. In each category, many different designs and styles are available. This section presents the basics and proceeds from there.

PLUS

Plus lenses are worn by patients who are farsighted (i.e., they can focus on objects far away but not on objects near them). The image in the patient's eye is falling behind the retina and needs to be brought forward to focus on the retina. Following are characteristics of a plus lens:

1. It is denoted by (+).
2. It magnifies images *(makes them larger)*.
3. Its design is *base to base* and it *converges* light (i.e., it bends the light in toward the middle, bringing the image forward to focus on the retina).
4. Because the image follows the apex of a lens, when a patient turns his or her head, the object being viewed seems to move away from the center. This is called *against motion*.
5. The greater the vertex distance *(farther away from the eye)*, the *stronger* the power of the lens.
6. The lens is thicker in the middle and thinner on the edges.

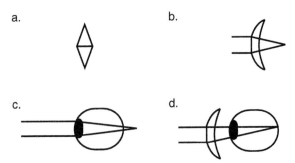

Figure 2-25 Plus lens design. **A,** Basic prism design. **B,** Actual view. **C,** View without lens. **D,** View with lens correction.

MINUS

Minus lenses are worn by patients who are nearsighted (i.e., they can focus on images near them but not on objects far away). The image in the patient's eye is falling in front of the retina and needs to be pushed back to focus on the retina. Following are characteristics of a minus lens:

1. It is denoted by (–).
2. It minifies images *(makes them smaller)*.
3. Its design is *apex to apex* and it *diverges* light (i.e., it bends the light away from the middle).
4. Because the image follows the apex of a lens, when a patient turns his or her head, the object being viewed seems to move with the center. This is called *with motion*.
5. The greater the vertex distance *(the farther away from the eye)*, the *weaker* the power of the lens.
6. The lens is thinner in the middle and thicker on the edges.

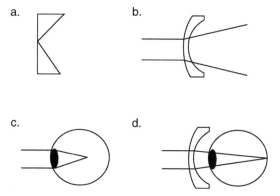

FIGURE 2-26 Minus lens design. **A,** Basic prism design. **B,** Actual view. **C,** View without lens. **D,** View with lens correction.

Astigmatism   The condition of having two focal points in the eye. (This is common.) It is a result of the shape of the eye *(like a football)* and/or the shape of the cornea *(having hills and valleys)*. The cornea has two different curves instead of one. The written prescription will have a cylinder and an axis.

Rx   An abbreviation for the word *prescription*. People commonly use the term *Rx* rather than write out or even say the whole word, *prescription*.

Sphere (Sph)   The base power of the lens. It has a singular curve on the front and back surface of the lens.

Cylinder (Cyl)   The secondary power in the lens to correct astigmatism. The front surface of the lens has one curve and the back surface has two different curves. The cylinder always has an axis and is always 90 degrees away from the location of the sphere.

Axis   The location of the cylinder. Its measurement is numbered from 0 to 180 degrees.

Add   The additional power added to the lens to magnify for reading. This prescription can be used for bifocals and trifocals. These patients have *presbyopia*.

Distance Vision   Any objects to be focused on beyond the length of the arms *(far away)*.

Intermediate Vision   Any objects to be focused on between the elbow and tip of the hand, usually between 18 and 36 inches from the face *(arm's length)*.

Near Vision   Any objects to be focused on between the tip of the nose to 12 or 18 inches from the face *(reading distance)*.

Peripheral Vision   The vision on the sides, up, and down when one is looking straight ahead *(out of the corner of the eye)*.

OD (Oculus Dexter)   Right eye.

OS (Oculus Sinister)   Left eye.

OU (Oculus Uterque)   Both eyes.

PD (Pupillary Distance)   The distance from center of one pupil to the center of the other pupil.

Monocular PD (Mono PD)   Separate measurement for each eye, taken from the center of the pupil to the center of the bridge of the nose. It is the most accurate PD measurement for making lenses, and is written as 31OD 32OS.

Binocular PD   Measurement of both eyes, taken from the center of one pupil to the center of the other pupil. It is the most common PD measurement taken, and is written as 63OU. It is usually referred to as simply *PD*.

Far PD   The measurement taken when the eyes are positioned to see straight ahead and are focused on an object in the distance. It is also referred to as the *distance PD*.

Near PD   The measurement taken when the eyes are positioned to see up close and are focused on an object within 18 inches of the front of the face. It is normally figured by measuring the far PD and then subtracting 3. Some opticians also use the following guideline to figure the number to subtract from the far PD:

Far PD	Subtract
≤59	2
60-66	3
≥67	4

You should use the method that is preferred in your clinic. *All methods are acceptable.*

Decentration The distance that the ocular center of the lens is set from the geometric center of the lens. The following formula is used to calculate the amount of decentration per eye or lens:

A measurement + DBL measurement − Patient's PD ÷ 2

For example, if the patient's PD is 63 and he is in a 50 − 18 eye-size frame, how far in should the decentration be set?

$$50 + 18 − 63 = 5$$
$$5 ÷ 2 = 2.5 \text{ mm set in per eye}$$

OC (Ocular Center) The point on the lens through which light passes without being bent. The centers must be aligned over the patient's pupils for the best vision to be achieved.

OC Ht (Ocular Center Height) The measurement from the farthest bottom inside edge of the frame to the center of the pupil when eyes are focused straight ahead.

Seg Ht (Segment Height) The height of the segment for bifocal, trifocal, and progressive lenses. It is measured from the line of the segment to the farthest bottom inside edge of the frame.

Seg Drop (Segment Drop) The distance down from the geometric center at which the bifocal line should be set. The following formula is used to calculate the seg drop:

B measurement ÷ 2 − Seg ht

For example, if the B measurement of patient's frame is 50 and the seg ht you measured is 18, what would the seg drop be?

$$50 ÷ 2 = 25$$
$$25 − 18 = 7\text{-mm drop from the center of the frame}$$

Edge Thickness The thickness of the outer edge of the lens.

CT (Center Thickness) The thickness in the center of the lens. All minus lenses have a set center thickness depending on what type of material is used. Following are some of the center thickness measurements for minus lenses in different materials:

Plastic   2.2 mm
Polycarbonate 1.5 or 1.0 mm
High index   1.0 mm
All safety   3.0 mm

> OSHA Standards require that all safety lenses be used only with
> safety frames and that all safety frames have safety lenses.

Plus lenses vary in center thickness because of the prescription. The stronger the prescription, the thicker the middle is going to be.

Bevel   The humped piece of the lens that fits in the groove of the frame. *A rimless frame has a groove.*

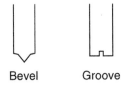

Bevel   Groove

FIGURE **2-27** Bevel and groove.

TYPES OF LENS MATERIALS

Plastic   Lens made from a CR-39 polymer, which is the most common material used. Sometimes people refer to plastic lenses as *CR-39* instead of as plastic. This material allows good optics and does not scratch easily. In addition, tints are easily applied to these lenses, and the tints can be lightened or darkened by the laboratory without causing damage to the lenses. All lens styles are available in plastic, and any coating can be applied to plastic. It is versatile, has a 1.53 index of refraction, and is available in 70-, 75-, and 80-mm blanks.

Polycarbonate   Lense made from a polycarbonate polymer. People usually refer to this material as *poly*. It is one of the thinnest, lightest materials on the market. It is impact resistant; however, the optics are not as good as those from plastic lenses. Visibility tends to be slightly distorted around the edges as the prescription strength, and thus the thickness of the lens, increases. Polycarbonate scratches easily and is difficult to tint. Tints do not darken as much as they do on plastic. In addition, lightening or darkening the tints on these lenses sometimes causes damage to the lenses or changes their color. Polycarbonate lenses may "shrink" in very cold temperatures. They can also expand, crack, and/or split in hot temperatures (e.g., being left in the car on a summer day). Polycarbonate has a 1.60 index of refraction (1.66 and higher indices are available), and is available in 70-, 75-, and 80-mm blanks.

Glass Lens made from glass; it is twice as heavy as a normal plastic lens. It has the best optics (i.e., there is little distortion in the lens). It has to be treated against shattering before it can be used by the patient. It can shatter, but it is difficult to scratch. Tints may be added; however, they are permanent. You *cannot* lighten or darken a tint on glass; a new lens must be made. Glass has a 1.55 index of refraction, and is available in 70- and 75-mm blanks.

High Index Lens made from a plastic material but at a higher refractive index than CR-39 polymer plastic, which makes it thinner and lighter, like polycarbonate. Its optics are comparable with plastic, it scratches easily, and tints are easily applied. However, much like with polycarbonate, when tints are lightened or darkened on high index lenses, they are sometimes discolored and the lenses may be damaged. As with poly, this material has a 1.60 index of refraction (1.66 and higher indices are available), and is available in 70-, 75-, and 80-mm blanks.

Index of refraction refers to the density of the material and its ability to refract *(bend)* light. The higher the index, the thinner the lens will be.

> The *blank size* is the size of the lens (in millimeters) before it is cut down to the measurements, size, and shape of the frame. The blank size used is determined by the frame size, the patient's pupillary measurements, and the prescription.

TYPES OF LENS STYLES

Single Vision Lens with one prescription, for either distance, intermediate, or near vision.

Bifocal Lens with two prescriptions, for distance and near vision or for intermediate and near vision. Bifocals are available in many different styles: ST 25, ST 28, ST 35, ST 45, round seg 22, round seg 24, round seg 28, executive, progressive addition lens (PAL), and lenticular 28 (used for patients with aphakia). The suggested minimal segment height for any bifocal is 11 to 12 mm. This allows adequate reading area.

Trifocal Lens with three different prescriptions, distance, intermediate, and near vision. Trifocals come in many different styles: 7×28, 8×35, 10×35, 14×35, executive, and PAL. The suggested minimal segment height for any lined trifocal is 18 to 19 mm. This allows adequate room for the reading area and the intermediate area.

ST (Straight Top) Lens with a straight top. This may also be written as FT (flat top). The number that follows ST or FT is the width of the bifocals in millimeters.

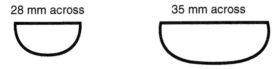

FIGURE **2-28** Lenses with straight tops.

Executive Lens on which the line for the bifocal or trifocal goes all the way across. It is thicker than most lenses because it is made by gluing the lenses together. It is also referred to as the *Franklin style*, because Benjamin Franklin invented it.

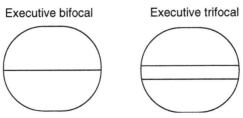

FIGURE **2-29** Executive lenses.

7 × 28 Lens that is named for its measurements. The *7* stands for the depth (in millimeters) of the trifocal segment (the intermediate) and the *28* stands for the width (in millimeters) of segment. The same can be applied to the 8 × 35, 10 × 35, and 14 × 35. You will not see the 10 × 35 or the 14 × 35 styles often.

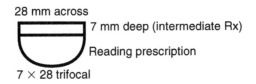

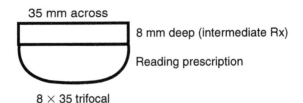

FIGURE **2-30** Straight-top trifocal lenses.

Progressive Addition Lens (PAL) The design of the lens. The front design on the lens is such that the prescription slowly changes from the distance Rx to the near Rx as the patient's focus moves down the lens with minimal head movement. This lens is most commonly referred to as the *invisible bifocal*, because you will not see any actual lines. However, you will see what are called *watermarks* on the lens. The lens will have two circles, crosses, stars, diamonds, arrows (or whatever symbol the manufacturer has chosen), and two numbers below one of the symbols to indicate the add power of the lens, as well as an emblem of some sort to identify the type of progressive lens and its manufacturer. Your laboratory should have a progressive lens identifier pamphlet.

The suggested minimal segment height for any progressive lens is 21 to 22 mm. You should check with your laboratory or supervisor, because progressive lens technology is rapidly advancing to allow for lower segment heights. The segment height is taken at the distance because there is a crosshair that is used as a reference point for verifying the prescription and in the layout process. The midrange and reading prescriptions are a standard length away from the distance. Those measurements have been calculated and set into the lens by the manufacturer. The segment height varies between each manufacturer and lens style, usually by only a few millimeters, but it can make the difference in whether the lens can fit in a frame or whether a patient can see as naturally as possible.

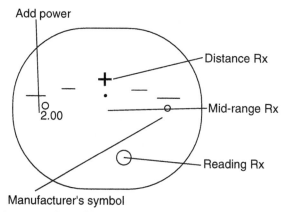

FIGURE 2-31 Progressive addition lens (PAL) blank.

LENS COATINGS AND EXTRAS

Tint The coloring of the lens. Many different colors and shades are available (e.g., gray, brown, green, pink-rose, blue, yellow, or combinations of any of these colors). The shades are available from a very light to a dark sunglasses tint. The different shades of color are labeled by numbers or percentages (e.g., gray #1, gray #2, gray #3, gray #4, with #1 being the lightest, or gray 10%, gray 30%, gray 80%, and so on, with 10% being the lightest). The percentage indicates the amount of light that is being blocked. Either method of labeling the shades of color is acceptable.

- Tint on *plastic lenses* can be lightened or darkened. Darkening the tint on an old pair of plastic lenses tends to show the scratches and sometimes, depending on how old the lenses are, it may ruin the lenses.
- Tint on *glass lenses* is permanent. If the patient wants to change the tint in any way, new lenses have to be made.
- Tint on *polycarbonate lenses* can be lightened and darkened, but you do not want to change the tint on the same pair of lenses too many times, because you chance ruining the lenses.
- Tint can be applied over the whole lens *(solid tint)* or the tint can be darker on the top and fade to clear at the bottom *(gradient tint)*. Tints *do not* change from light to dark when going from inside to outside. Lenses are tinted in the laboratory and the process is much like dying eggs. The longer the lens is left in the dye, the darker it gets.

> All tints inhibit vision somewhat. The darker the tint, the more the vision will be affected, especially if the patient wears sunglasses tints indoors or in dim lighting.

Transitions III   A plastic lens that changes from a light or almost clear tint when the patient is indoors to a darker tint when he or she goes outdoors. It blocks UV rays and is a blue-gray or brown color. The changing process results from the exposure to UV rays. This lens is sensitive to heat and cold. It does not change as well in higher temperatures (hot summer) or when the patient is riding in the car, wearing a hat, or standing in the shade, because the lens is blocked from UV exposure. This lens gets darker in cold temperatures (winter weather). Therefore if the patient works in a cold place or someplace where the air-conditioner is kept low, the tint will always be slightly darker than usual. The lens sometimes has difficulty activating the changing process for the first couple of days, because it needs a day or two of exposure to UV light to lighten and darken quickly. This lens is also referred to as *T3* for short.

Transitions XrtActive   Lens that has the same properties as the Transitions III, except the XrtActive is *darker*, both indoors and outdoors. It is also referred to as *TX* or *Trans Xtra*.

Photogray Extra   A glass lens that changes from a light tint indoors to a darker tint outdoors. The lens blocks UV rays and is sensitive to temperatures, in the same manner as the Transitions lens. This lens also needs a few days' exposure to UV light for the changing process to activate so that the lens turns quickly. It is referred to as *PGX* or simply *Photogray*.

UV   A clear coating added to the lens to filter out UV rays. This helps slow the development of cataracts. Over a long period, the lens becomes slightly yellowed from absorbing UV.

UV 500   A bright yellow-brown coating that filters out UV rays. Some laboratories call it a *blue-blocker tint*. It decreases glare, and some people like it for hunting or the shooting range. Another color tint may be applied over UV 500 to change the color a little; however, the yellow color remains underneath whatever tint is put on top.

Hard Coat   A clear coating applied to the lenses to protect them against scratches. The lenses will eventually scratch; the coating only makes them more difficult to scratch. A hard coat is also referred to as a *scratch coat*. It can be compared with the clear gloss coat on a car. The coating protects the lens (or car) from surface scratches, but it does not prevent scratches from ever happening.

ARC   ARC is an *antireflective coating* that eliminates reflections on the front and back surface of the lens. It sharpens the patient's vision, because more light is able to pass through the lens instead of being bounced off the lens. ARC allows approximately 98% of light to pass through the lens. It also blocks UV rays (not as well as the UV coating, but it does absorb a good amount). It is highly recommended that an ARC be applied for the following patients:

1. Patients who wear polycarbonate lenses, because these lenses are quite dense and do not allow light to pass through easily
2. Patients who have trouble driving at night because of the reflections of oncoming cars and overhead lights
3. Patients who do a lot of computer work

Polarized   A filter that is sandwiched inside the lens to cut glare. It is available in different shades of gray, brown, and green, labeled as #1, #2, and #3, with #1 being the lightest and #3 being the darkest. The most common shade sold is the #3 sunglasses tint. This lens is recommended for patients who do a lot of fishing, skiing, or any outdoor sport where glare can be a problem.

Roll   Process by which the edge of the lens is flattened so that it does not appear as thick from the side. It does tend to leave a "ring" around the lens that is visible when the lens is viewed from the front, depending on how much of the lens is rolled.

Polish   Process by which the lens is buffed on the side (where the bevel or groove is) to make it appear clear and less noticeable. When the patient looks through the lens, he or she will notice some reflections for the first few days. This goes away in time.

Mirror Coating   The silver coating applied to the lenses of some sunglasses so that when they are viewed from the front, they look like mirrors. This coating is not applied often, and when it is, it is usually a very expensive process.

> To learn more about coatings and tints, please read the textbook, *Professional Dispensing for Opticianry* (Opticians Association of America Staff, 1996).

BASIC WRITTEN CONTACT LENS PRESCRIPTION

Name:___*Lily Smith*___   Date:___*11-15-01*___

Address:_____

OD_____*−2.50*____*8.6*_____*14.0*_____

OS_____*−3.50*____*8.6*_____*14.0*_____

Comments ___*Acuvue 2 Disp   2 wk wear*___

Dr. *Mike Jeckle OD*_____

Exp._*11-15-02*_____

FIGURE 2-32 Basic written contact lens prescription. *14.0*, The diameter of the lens; *2-week wear*, Tells you the length of time the patient wears one pair of contact lenses; *−2.50 and −3.50*, Power of the contact lens (if it were a Toric lens, it would have a cylinder power and axis like glasses); *8.6*, The base curve of the lens; *Acuvue 2*, The brand name of the contact lenses to order; *OD*, Right eye; *OS*, Left eye.

> All contact lens prescriptions must have a doctor's signature and an expiration date. Always check with the prescribing doctor if you have any questions or doubts about the prescription.

CONTACT LENSES

Base Curve (BC)   The curve of the front surface of the contact lens; written as 8.3, 8.4, 8.5, 8.6, 8.7, 8.8, 9.0, 9.1, and so on.

Diameter (Dia)   The size (in millimeters) of the contact lens; written as 13.5, 14.0, 14.5, 15.0, and so on.

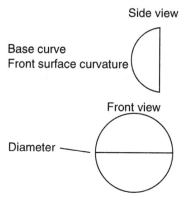

FIGURE 2-33 Base curve and diameter.

"K" readings   The measurements taken off the front surface of the cornea to determine what the curvature (base curve) of the lens needs to be.

Toric   Lenses that corrects for astigmatism. The cornea has more than one curve on its surface, so the contact lenses need to have more than one curve to compensate for this.

Soft Lens   Lens made of plastic. It changes shape to fit the shape of the cornea. It can flip inside and out. The contact lens looks like a bowl with the edges pointing to the inside when it is right side out. It looks like a saucer with the edges flared out when it is inside out. It requires a lot of moisture. This lens is very porous and can tear easily. In addition, the lens traps a lot of dirt in its pours, which the eye sloughs off during the day. This is the reason it is so important to clean soft lenses often. Several different types of soft contact lenses are available (e.g., daily wear, extended wear, disposable, planned replacement). Each of these names refers to how long the lens may be worn without being removed.

Hard Lens   Lens that is quite stiff and is made of plastic. The shape of the cornea will change to fit the contact lens. A hard lens does *not* flip inside and out. It can break, chip, and/or crack. Most hard lenses are worn the same way: worn during the day and taken out at night to be cleaned and to let the eyes rest. Hard lenses are also very porous and able to trap the dirt the eye leaves behind. Enzymatic cleaner is used once a week to remove built-up deposits that the daily cleaning did not remove from the lenses. Because the lenses are hard, the patient literally develops a callus on the inside of the eyelid because of the constant rubbing during blinking. This callus is not harmful, the patient simply does not feel the contact lens anymore. Hard lenses are also called *rigid gas permeable (RGP) lenses*.

TYPES OF SOFT LENSES

Daily Wear (DW)   A soft lens that is worn all day and taken out at night to be cleaned and to let the eyes rest. It is one of the "thickest" types of soft contact lenses. It does not allow a lot of oxygen to pass through, therefore it is recommended that the patient not sleep in these contact lenses. They dry out, stick to the patient's eyes, and become difficult to remove.

Extended Wear (EW)   A soft lens that may be worn for 3 to 4 days, and even up to a week at a time, without having to be taken out. It is a thinner lens that allows more oxygen to pass through, so it may be slept in. It needs to be removed once a week for an enzymatic cleaning to remove all deposits from the lens. It is also called a *frequent wear (FW) lens*.

Disposable   A soft lens that is generally worn for 2 to 4 weeks at a time and is removed only once a week to be cleaned of deposits. After 2 to 4 weeks of wear, the lenses are thrown away and a fresh new pair is put in.

Planned Replacement   A soft lens that is worn for 3 to 4 months at a time. It is removed once a week for a cleaning. After 3 to 4 months of wear, the lenses are thrown away and a fresh new pair is put in.

The length of time a patient wears a soft lens is always determined by the doctor. Following are some of the factors considered when fitting a patient for lenses:

1. The amount of deposits that builds up in the eyes
2. The amount of tears the eyes produce
3. The amount of oxygen the eyes need
4. The manner in which the patient cares for his or her lenses (cleaning and handling)

Handling Tint A light tint (generally blue or green) put on the lens so that the contact lens may be seen easily in solutions. It does not affect the color of the eye. It is also called a *visitint*.

Colored Lenses Soft lenses that are tinted different colors to either change the natural color of the eye or enhance the natural color of the eye.

Opaque A tint put on the lens that is dark enough to change the color of the eye. It is used mostly for patients with dark-colored eyes, but it also can be used on patients with light-colored eyes.

Enhancer A tint put on the lens that is dark enough to change the color of the eye for patients with light eyes or is used only to enhance the color of dark or light eyes.

Bifocal Contact Lenses Contact lenses for patients who have presbyopia. Both focal points are corrected with only one lens. One bifocal is designed with "rings" that alternate for distance correction and near correction. Other designs are much like the progressive lenses for glasses and some look like a lined bifocal lens for glasses.

Monovision Contact Lenses Contact lenses for people who have presbyopia. Two different lenses are worn. One lens corrects for distance vision and one lens corrects for near vision. It takes a while for the patient to become accustomed to these lenses, because the eyes now act separately from each other instead of together as they normally would.

CONTACT LENS INSTRUCTION ON WEAR AND CARE

When you are teaching patients how to wear and care for their contact lenses, the most important and first thing you must always do is *wash your hands*. You must also emphasize the importance of handwashing to all patients. The following is a guideline on the instruction of inserting and removing contact lenses. Remember, you will end up adopting your own style. In addition, check with your trainer or supervisor to see whether you will be performing this duty. Not every optician is expected to teach patients contact lens wear and care.

INSERTION OF CONTACT LENSES

1. Wash your hands. Make sure the patient washes his or her hands.
2. Show the patient how to situate the lens on the tip of the index (pointer) finger. Make sure the contact lens is wet and the finger is dry. This helps when putting the contact lens on the eye. If the finger is wet, the lens tends to stick to the finger and not adhere to the cornea.
3. Make sure the contact lens is right side out. It looks like a bowl when it is right side out and it looks like a saucer when it is wrong side out. If

you are not sure whether the lens is the right side out, flip it a few times to see the difference. It is also helpful for the patient to see this. You will not have to do any of this with hard contact lenses. They *do not* flip in and out. They are hard and keep their shape.

Right side out (correct)

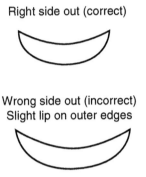

Wrong side out (incorrect)
Slight lip on outer edges

FIGURE **2-34** Contact lens sides.

4. With the hand that *is not* holding the lens, the patient should place his or her finger on the eyelid right above the lashes and roll the finger up to the bone surrounding the eye.
5. With the hand that is holding the contact lens, the patient should pull down the bottom eyelid the same way he or she did the top eyelid.
6. Instruct the patient to keep both eyes open wide the whole time. If one eye is shut, the other will also try to shut.
7. The patient should gently place the lens directly over the iris. Sometimes this requires a gentle "push"; the key word here is *gentle*. Remind the patient that he or she does not want to damage the eye.
8. Instruct the patient to *slowly* draw the finger back, but to not let go of the eyelids.
9. Ask the patient to look down while keeping his or her eyelids open.
10. He or she should now close the eyelids slowly and deliberately.
11. Using a tissue or the fingertip, gently tap the lid to make sure all of the air bubbles are gone.
12. Instruct the patient to roll the eye around.
13. He or she can now open the eyes, and the lens should be in place.

> Teaching contact lens insertion requires a lot of practice and patience. Be prepared to sit down with a new contact lens patient for about an hour. In general, these patients will blink a lot and their eyes will water a lot. It is also normal for their eyes to become blood shot. New contact lens wearers should be forewarned about these common reactions before they come in for their appointment.
> Remember, hard contact lenses are easier to insert than soft contact lenses are; however, hard lenses are not as easily removed.

REMOVAL OF CONTACT LENSES

For Soft Contact Lenses   Instruct the patient to open the eye just as he or she did with the insertion of the lens. Using the thumb and the forefinger, the patient should gently grab the lens at the outer edges, pinch it together, and pull it out. This also takes some practice.

For Hard Contact Lenses   To remove a hard lens, the patient needs to break the suction between the eye and the lens. Instruct the patient in the following two ways of doing this:

1. Open the eye as wide as possible.
2. Place a finger at the outer edge of the eye where the top lid and the bottom lid meet.
3. Pull back as tight possible and blink hard.
4. Holding the other hand below the eye, catch the lens.

Tell the patient that he or she can break the suction another way:

- With a finger, push the bottom lid right up to the edge of the lens and look down.

The patient may find another way that works for him or her. As long as the contact lens is removed and cleaned without damage, it is all right. The patient must be able to insert and remove the contact by himself or herself before leaving your office.

When you are teaching patients about wear and care of contact lenses, always remember to make sure the storage and cleaning solutions are set up, ready to use, or nearby. *Do not* use the fingernails for insertion or removal of contact lenses. Patients with long fingernails need to be aware of this. They must learn to use the finger itself when touching their eyes. Some doctors may even advise these patients to cut their fingernails, because dirt can become trapped under the fingernails and contaminate the lens and the eyes.

CLEANING

Many different cleaning solutions arc available for the many different cleaning needs. Cleaning solutions and needs vary because of the many types of soft contact lenses and wearing times. Please check with your trainer or supervisor to find out which cleaning solutions are carried in your office and to learn how each one is used. In addition, check with the doctor to see which type of solutions he or she prefers to use for each type of contact lens.

All hard contact lenses need to be cleaned daily, stored overnight, and cleaned with enzymes once a week to remove the deposits the daily cleaning did not remove.

To learn more about contact lenses, please read the textbook, *Contact Lenses: Procedures and Techniques* (GE Lowther, C Snyder, 1992), available from Elsevier.

LEVEL 2 ASSESSMENT

1. True or False: It is more appropriate to say "My next available appointment with Dr. Smith is..." rather than "The doctor can't see you then."

2. When making an appointment for a patient, it is important to know:
   A. How much he or she likes you
   B. What sports he or she plays
   C. The reason for the appointment
   D. If he or she has any nicknames

3. The pupil is the:
   A. Opening in the middle of the eye
   B. Back of the eye
   C. Black ring around the iris
   D. Colored part of the eye

4. The retina is the:
   A. Colored part of the eye
   B. Opening in the middle of the eye
   C. Back of the eye
   D. Black ring around the iris

5. The rods and cones are located in the:
   A. Optic nerve
   B. Macula
   C. Pupil
   D. Choroid

6. How many muscles control eye movement?
   A. 4
   B. 6
   C. 5
   D. 3

7. Presbyopia is the:
   A. Ability to see far away
   B. Loss of ability to accommodate for near vision
   C. Ability to see close up
   D. Vision to the side

8. How many different types of astigmatism are there?
   A. 5
   B. 4
   C. 6
   D. 2

9. The condition of the patient not having equal amounts of correction from one eye to the next is called:
   A. Emmetropia
   B. Ametropia
   C. Anisometropia
   D. Amblyopia

10. The condition of fluid building up inside the eye is called:
    A. Strabismus
    B. Hyperopia
    C. Glaucoma
    D. Diplopia
11. Light travels at what speed?
    A. 184,000 miles/sec
    B. 186,000 miles/sec
    C. 186,000 miles/hr
    D. 185,000 miles/hr
12. Refractive index refers to:
    A. Density
    B. Thickness
    C. Angle of refraction
    D. Distance
13. Which of the following *does not* effect the power of the lens?
    A. Curvature
    B. Density
    C. Distance
    D. Angle of light
14. True or False: The thicker the lens is, the greater its ability to bend light.
15. What is the A measurement of a frame?
    A. The diagonal measurement
    B. The vertical measurement
    C. The horizontal measurement
    D. The distance between the pupils
16. Where on the frame would you find the manufacturer and the name (or style number) of the frame?
    A. On the bridge
    B. Temple tip
    C. Eye wire
    D. On inside of the temple
17. Which one is *not* a type of frame material?
    A. Pure gold
    B. Titanium
    C. Optyl
    D. Metal
18. Pantoscopic tilt is:
    A. The lack of ability to accommodate for reading
    B. The angle of a frame: the frame is closer to the face at the top
    C. How the patient holds his or her head
    D. The angle of the frame: the frame is closer to the face at the bottom

19. Plus lenses are worn by patients who are:
    A. Emmetropic
    B. Farsighted
    C. Esophoric
    D. Nearsighted
20. The sphere is the:
    A. Location of the cylinder
    B. Magnifying power of the lens
    C. Base power of the lens
    D. Secondary power to correct astigmatism
21. Name four basic lens styles.
22. Name four basic lens materials.
23. If a patient complains that his or her nose pads are causing discomfort, you should:
    A. Loosen the temples of the frame
    B. Loosen the nose pads of the frame
    C. Give the frame more pantoscopic tilt
    D. Bend the front of the frame
24. If the patient complains that one side of the frame is closer to his or her face than the other, it means:
    A. The frame has too much pantoscopic tilt
    B. The temple tips are too long
    C. The temples are shifted
    D. The frame has too much retroscopic tilt
25. The tint on plastic lenses:
    A. Does not change when the patient goes from inside to outside
    B. Changes slightly when the patient goes from inside to outside
    C. Is permanent and can never be lightened or darkened
    D. Is a clear coating that filters out UV rays
26. The difference between a transition lens and a Photogray lens is:
    A. One changes tint, the other one does not
    B. One is five times darker than the other one
    C. One is glass, the other one is plastic
    D. One has no reflections, the other one does
27. If the patient does not want the sides of his or her lenses to be too noticeable, what should be done to the lenses?
    A. They should be polished.
    B. A hard coating should be applied.
    C. A mirror coating should be applied.
    D. An ARC should be applied.
28. The base curve of a contact lens is the:
    A. Correction for astigmatism
    B. Size of the contact

    C. Measurement of the eyeball

    D. Curvature of the front surface of the lens

29. True or False: Disposable contact lenses are generally worn for 2 weeks and then thrown away.

30. The most important rule of inserting contact lenses is:

    A. Hold your elbows high

    B. Wash your hands

    C. Close the lids quickly

    D. Make sure the fingertips are wet

LEVEL 3

Optician Apprentice

OBJECTIVES

- Continue your education as an optician.
- Increase the amount of one-on-one work you do with patients, fitting glasses and filling prescriptions.

TASKS TO MASTER

- Learn **more about lenses**
- Learn about **choosing lenses**
- Learn about **face shapes**
- Learn about **frame styling**
- Begin **taking measurements**
- Familiarize yourself with the **lensometer**
- Learn about **transposing**

You should be closely supervised while you learn all of these tasks, until you have mastered this level.

LEVEL 3 SCHEDULE

In Level 3, you should be doing most of your daily tasks on your own. Everything you do should be double-checked by your trainer or another optician. An assessment will be given to check your progress.

LEVEL 3 OPTICIAN APPRENTICE

Task

Stage 1

Read assigned material: *More About Lenses*	
Read assigned material: *Choosing Lenses*	
Answer the phones and make appointments	
Start fitting patients with frames	

Stage 2

Read assigned material: *Face Shapes*	
Read assigned material: *Frame Styling*	
Continue fitting patients with frames	
Continue answering the phones and making appointments	

Stage 3

Read assigned material: *Taking Measurements*	
Read assigned material: *Lensometer*	
Practice using the lensometer	
Continue answering the phones and making appointments	
Continue fitting patients with frames	
Start taking measurements on patients	

Stage 4

Read assigned material: *Transposing*	
Use the lensometer and practice transposing a prescription	
Continue answering the phones and making appointments	
Continue fitting patients with frames	
Continue taking measurements on patients	

Stage 5

Continue using the lensometer and practicing transposing prescriptions	
Continue answering the phones and making appointments	
Continue using the lensometer and practicing transposing prescriptions	
Do some adjustments and repairs on patients' glasses	
Continue fitting patients with frames	
Continue taking measurements on patients	
Complete *Level 3 Assessment* and ask your trainer to review it	

MORE ABOUT LENSES

PRISM

Prism   A method of redirecting light. The term *prism* will now be used in a context different from the context in which it was used previously. *Prism* now refers to the ocular center not being placed directly over the pupil. Prism can be caused by moving a lens "off center," which means moving the optical center. When the term *prism* is used in optical, it usually refers to the prism diopter, not the actual wedge. Prism can be either prescribed or unwanted.

Prism Diopter   Unit of measure denoting how far the optical center is displaced from where it should be.

Prescribed Prism   Prism that the doctor has determined is necessary for the patient. The doctor most commonly prescribes a prism because the patient's eye muscles are pulling the eye one way and they need to be trained to pull the eye forward.

Unwanted Prism   Prism that the doctor did not prescribe that is found in glasses. Unwanted prism is the result of the optical centers being placed somewhere other than over the pupil. With unwanted prism, the patient feels a pulling sensation.

If the pupillary distance (PD) is not made to the patient's measurements (the PD is off), or if the ocular heights differ from one eye to the next, there will be a prismatic effect. To determine the amount of prismatic effect the glasses may have, opticians use a formula known as *Prentice's Rule*.

Prentice's Rule

$$\text{Prism diopters} = c \times F$$

where

Prism diopters (prismatic effect) = Amount of unwanted prism in the lens
c = Amount (in centimeters) the PD is off (i.e., decentration)
F = Refractive power of the lens (in diopters)
For example, when you examine a pair of glasses, you find the PD is off by 5 mm. The prescription is a +4.00. How much prismatic effect will this cause?

$$\text{Prism diopters} = 0.5 \times 4.00$$

$$= 2.00 \text{ diopters of prism}$$

The answer is 2 diopters of prismatic effect.

There are four basic directions of prism: base up, base down, base in, and base out.

> The light is always bent toward the *base* (thickest end) of the prism, making the object appear to be displaced toward the *apex* (thinnest end) of the prism. Keep this in mind—it will help you visualize prism direction better.

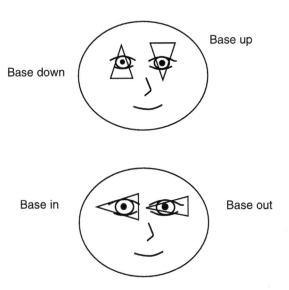

Figure 3-1 A basic view of base directions. The base is the thickest part of the lens.

Compounding Prism   Using prism in two different directions to create more prism effect. This is sometimes done to split the prism between the eyes so that one eye does not have to do all the work; thus the patient can adapt easier to the prescription.

Compounding Situations
Base in and base in
Base out and base out
Base up and base down

Canceling Prism   A method of reducing the effect of the prism. The eyes move in the same direction, so the prism has no effect.

Canceling Situations
Base up and base up
Base down and base down
Base in and base out

Slab-Off   A method of redirecting light in a lens, usually used for patients whose prescriptions differ greatly from one eye to the other (usually 2 diopters or more difference) (e.g., OD –5.50 –0.25 × 97 OS +0.75 × –0.50 85). Because of the difference in the power of each lens, the images appear to be in two different places and the patient may see double. Therefore to get both of the images in approximately the same place so that the patient no longer sees double, the doctor may ask for slab-off. It is done by cutting off a calculated amount of the lower portion of the lens. (All of these calculations are done by the laboratory.) This causes prism and redirects the image. The lens looks as if a line goes all the way across it. The line is not as noticeable as the line of a bifocal, but it is visible. If you need to know on which lens the line will appear, the rule is that slab-off is done on the lens with the most minus or least plus (depending on the prescription). Slab-off is commonly done on bifocal lenses, because the patient usually notices the image "jump" only when he or she looks through the bifocal. Slab-off is occasionally done on a single vision lens.

BASE CURVES

Lenses are made in quarter diopter powers. This means they progress as follows:

Spheres

Plano or 0.00   0.25 sphere   0.50 sphere   0.75 sphere   and so on

Cylinders

Plano –0.25 →	–0.25 → –0.5
Plano –0.50 →	–0.50 → –0.5
Plano –0.75 →	–0.75 → –0.5
Plano –1.00 →	–1.00 → –0.5

Base Curve   Measurement of the single curve on the front side of the lens (in diopters). The instrument used to measure the base curve is called the *lens clock;* it can measure the front and back curves.

Back Curve   The curve on the back side of the lens.

Spherical Lenses   Lenses that have a single curve on the front surface and one curve on the back surface. The prescription is written as a sphere only (e.g., OD –3.00 D sph OS –2.50 D sph).
   D sph means diopter sphere.

Cylindrical Lenses   Lenses that have one curve on the front side and two curves on the back side. This means that a cylindrical power has been ground into the back of the lens to correct for astigmatism. The two curves are 90 degrees away from each other. A cylindrical lens is in *minus cylinder* form. These lenses are sometimes referred to as *toric lenses*.

Minus Cylinder Form   The cylinder is ground into the back side of the lens (the two curves on the back of the lens). This is the reason the laboratory needs to know the prescription with the cylinder being in minus cylinder form and not in plus cylinder form (i.e., $-1.00 - 1.00 \times 90$ is minus cylinder form and $-2.00 + 1.00 \times 180$ is plus cylinder form).

Aspheric Lenses   Lenses that have more than one curve on the front side. The front surface of the lens has a central base curve and a series of different curves that move from the center of the lens to the edge, making a flatter and thinner lens. This design is used for all progressive lenses to achieve the no-line effect between the top prescription for distance vision and the bottom prescription for near vision. This design is also used to create a thinner lens for a heavy plus prescription. The different curves greatly affect the prescription.

Front and back curves directly affect each other. Each prescription has a recommended or standard base curve. Some laboratories use odd numbers and some use even numbers to denote the standard base curve. Base curves move in quarter diopters as power does. Following is a guideline for which base curves to use with which prescriptions. These may differ depending on the type of lens design or whether a special base curve is desired.

Prescription	Base Curve
−12.00 to −8.00	plano or 2 base
−8.00 to −2.00	2 base or 4 base
−2.00 to +2.00	6 base
+2.00 to +6.00	8 base
+6.00 to +11.00	10 base or 12 base

> For any prescription higher than +7.00, an aspheric lens is recommended.

The front and back curves help determine the lens power. The higher the plus power, the steeper the front curve is and the greater the base curve is. The higher the minus power, the flatter the front curve is and the lower the base curve is.

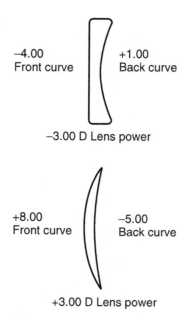

FIGURE 3-2 Minus and plus curves.

To calculate the power of the lens, add the measurements of the front and back curves.

−4.00 front curve	+8.00 front curve
(+) +1.00 back curve	(+) −5.00 back curve
−3.00 lens power	+3.00 lens power

To learn more about lenses, read the textbooks *Understanding Lens Surfacing* (CW Brooks, 1992) and *Professional Dispensing for Opticianry* (Opticians Association of America Staff, 1996), both available from Elsevier.

CHOOSING LENSES

Before choosing a frame, you should choose the lenses that best suit the patient's needs and wants. It is a tremendous help if you know what lenses the patient needs before you select a frame; however you are not always so lucky. The actual prescription is the first major factor in choosing lenses. The patient needs one of the following types of lenses: single vision lenses, bifocals, or trifocals. You should note any remarks made by the doctor. He or she has sometimes already talked to the patient and has recommended certain types of lenses.

When choosing a lens, you should consider the following:

1. *Lens material*—The prescription gives you a chance to offer the best lens material available. If the prescription is more than ±2.00 diopters, you

should offer a polycarbonate lens. Because of the safety factor of poly-carbonate lenses, they should be suggested for children and for patients who play sports. You should use caution with prescriptions below 2.00 diopters, because there is a risk that the lens edge will be too thin to fit inside the frame. Some patients may prefer to stay with plastic lens. You should always make the patient aware of the benefits and disadvantages of the lens material he or she has chosen. These are discussed in the section *Lenses* in Level 2.

2. *Type of lens*—What will be the main use of the glasses? Reading? Computer work? Playing sports? Driving? Everything from driving to reading? The answers to these questions will help you decide what type of lens the patient may need (e.g., single vision, lined bifocal, lined trifocal, progressive addition lens [PAL]). If the patient needs a bifocal or trifocal, you must ask whether he or she prefers a lined bifocal or trifocal or a no-line bifocal or trifocal. If the patient wants a lined bifocal or trifocal, you must then determine the size (e.g., ST 28, ST 35), depending on the amount of room he or she needs for his or her reading area. With the no-line bifocal, the patient receives the benefit of a trifocal, because the design of the lens already includes the midrange prescription. You will have to explain to the patient how to use the lenses he or she has chosen. *Lined bifocals* have a line so that the patient knows when the prescription changes from distance to reading. The patient will be able to simply lower his or her eyes to read or to do close-up work. In the same respect, he or she will not be able to read small print or to do near work when he or she is looking out the top of the glasses. The top prescription is for distance only. The patient will have to get used to the lens and its advantages. *Lined trifocals* are similar to lined bifocals except the trifocals have the intermediate prescription right above the reading prescription. The patient may have to lift his or her head slightly to look at something at arms' length to ensure that he or she is looking through the intermediate prescription. *Progressive addition lenses* do not have any lines that show the patient where the prescription changes. You should inform the patient that he or she will notice changes in the prescription when he or she moves his or her head up and down and from side to side. The up-and-down changes are from the prescription changing from distance to reading. The side-to-side changes are distortion on the edges resulting from the lens design.

3. *Light sensitivity*—Is the patient sensitive to light? Indoors? Outdoors? The answers to these questions help you decide whether the patient needs tints, Transition lenses, or even a second pair of prescription sunglasses. The patient may want some tint to help with glare. You should first ask the patient whether he or she wants a permanent tint (stays the same shade when he or she goes from inside to outside) or Transitions (changes shades when he or she goes from inside to outside). Then, you must determine which shade the patient prefers (darker or lighter). The

patient may want a clear pair of glasses for wearing inside and a pair of sunglasses for outside. You should always recommend a UV coating, because it acts like sunscreen for the eyes. It is a clear coating that filters out ultraviolet (UV) rays, which can cause damage to the eyes much like they do to the skin. If the patient chooses a Transition lens, you should always explain that the lens requires a few days' exposure to UV rays to become active. If the patient chooses any tints, you should inform him or her that when tints are worn indoors, they can inhibit vision (i.e., the patient might not see as clearly indoors with a tint).

4. *Night vision or computer work*—Does the patient have trouble with driving at night? Reflections from the computer? Reflections from the back of his or her glasses? This gives you the chance to offer an anti-reflective coating (ARC). ARC helps patients with driving at night; it also helps cut down on reflections during the day. The coating is put on both sides of the lens and allows 98% more light to pass through the lens than would pass through without ARC, resulting in crisper vision. You should explain to the patient that to clean a lens with an ARC, it is better to use a lens cleaning cloth and *not* paper towels or clothing. The patient must also be educated to not rub hard when cleaning a lens with an ARC, because this only smears the dirt and oils that are on the lens. It is easier to clean a lens with an ARC using light-pressure rubbing. In addition, you should inform the patient that he or she will more easily notice dirt on the lenses, because there are no reflections hiding the dirt.

The previous section presented the basic concerns you should think about when choosing a lens for a patient. You will find more options to explore with each patient, because all patients are unique and special.

Certain things *do* go together and certain things *do not* go together. Because there are always changes and breakthroughs in technology, please check with your laboratory to find out whether certain products are available or recommended.

Following are a few lens and frame characteristics that go together well:

1. *Polycarbonate and ARC*—Because polycarbonate is dense, the optics are not as good as they can be, because light is not allowed to pass through. The ARC allows more light to pass through the lens. The result is sharper, clearer vision. ARC is good on any lens for this reason.

2. *High plus lens and aspheric design*—The aspheric design flattens the front and back of the lens, which makes it thinner. The result is a happy patient. Remember, all PALs are already made on the aspheric design.

3. *High minus lens and polycarbonate*—You have two choices with a polycarbonate lens: One has a 1.5 center thickness and the other has a 1.0 center thickness. With a minus lens, the thinner the center thickness, the thinner the edge will be.

Following are a few lens and frame characteristics that do *not* go together well:

1. *High plus lens in a rimless frame* (the frame with fishing wire)—Because the edge of a plus lens is thin, there is not enough space to cut the groove in to hold the wire. The lens will chip and flake.
2. *High plus or high minus lens in a large frame* (e.g., 53 eye size and higher)—A high plus or high minus lens can be put in a large frame, but the lens ends up being very thick and heavy.
3. *High plus or high minus lens in a drill-mount frame*—The lens will be too thick to drill through to make it fit properly on the frame pieces, and in the event you are able to drill all the way through the lens, the frame will have to be bent to appear straight because of how the pieces rest against the steep curve on the back side of the lens. The result is a poor-fitting pair of glasses.

Remember, these are the basics of choosing a lens to suit the patient's lifestyle and prescription. You will adapt your own style and presentation the more you sell. You will also learn more options to explore with the more experience that you get and the more products that become available.

When using a large frame, it may be necessary to determine the size of the lens needed. This is usually done when you are trying to use a lens from your stock inventory. You will calculate the size by using the Minimum Blank Size (MBS) formula.

Minimum Blank Size (MBS)   The smallest-diameter lens that will fit into a chosen frame after it is cut out according to the frame measurements and the patient's measurements. For example, you have a patient who needs a single vision lens, and he chooses a large frame. His PD is average or small and you need to determine whether you have a large enough lens in stock or whether you have to order it. You can use one of the following equations to calculate the MBS.

$$\text{MBS} = \text{Frame PD} - \text{Patient's PD} + \text{ED measurement}$$

or

$$\text{MBS} = (\text{A measurement} + \text{DBL}) - \text{Patient's PD} + \text{ED measurement}$$

$$\text{MBS} = (56 + 18) - 63 + 61$$
$$= 74 - 63 + 61$$
$$= 11 + 61$$
$$= 72\text{-mm blank}$$

Most laboratories carry 75-mm semifinished blanks in stock, because this is usually the size that will cut out for most job orders.

FRAME STYLING

Choosing the lens first narrows down the choice of frame styles the patient may choose. If the patient has a bifocal lens, he or she will need a frame with enough depth to fit the bifocal. The thickness of the lens may rule out rimless or drill-mount frames.

When frame styling, you should first talk with the patient to determine the following information:

1. What purpose the glasses serve
   A. Does the patient wear the glasses full time (never taking them off)?
   B. Does the patient want a frame that will go with anything he or she wears?
   C. Does the patient wear the glasses only when working on the computer or doing close-up work?
   D. Does the patient wear the glasses only for backup when he or she is not wearing contact lenses?
   E. Does the patient want only sunglasses or does he or she want one clear pair of glasses and one pair of sunglasses?
2. What type of lifestyle the patient has
   A. Does the patient work on cars or outside, requiring a more durable frame?
   B. Is he or she involved in many sports?
   C. Does the patient work with children and need a flexible frame?
   D. Is the patient allergic to metal frames?

This information will help you determine what type of frame is best for the patient. Sometimes you have to explain to the patient that although a frame looks fashionable, it is not the best frame for his or her needs. The frame style needs to fit the patient's lifestyle.

Following are some factors to consider when choosing a frame for a patient:

1. *The frame shape*—You should first decide what shape face the patient has and then choose a frame that is the opposite shape. This balances the facial features. For example, if the patient has a round face, you should choose frames that are square or octagon. This will make the face appear thinner and less round. To begin, you should present four or five frames to the patient and narrow the selection to one or two. Then, you should present four or five more frames and narrow the selection to the two or three best frames of all the selections presented. The frame that is best for the patient is then chosen from this final selection. It will take several minutes of trying on frames and looking at every angle for the patient to make a final decision. Remember to treat the patient as though he or she is one of your best friends. You do not want him or her going out of your store with unsuitable glasses and telling everyone where he or she got them.
2. *Color of the frame*—You should try to pick a color that complements the patients' skin tone and hair color. Some patients like the frame to match the jewelry they wear. They think of their glasses as an accessory. When it comes to color, remember, darker skin tones need darker or

neutral frame colors, and lighter skin tones need lighter or neutral frame colors. The patient should try on frames in several colors. It will be apparent which colors work and which ones do not.

3. *Eye size*—Currently, the fashion is smaller frames; however, you want the patient to have enough room to see out of the frame. The temples of the frame should go straight back. If they bend in toward the head, the frame is too big. If they bend out away from the head, the frame is too small. With regard to the depth (up and down) of the eye wire, the top of the frame should line up with or fall just below the eyebrows. (The patient will tell you whether he or she has a preference.) The bottom of the frame should fall approximately half way down the length of the nose. This helps ensure that the frame does not touch the patient's cheeks, even when he or she smiles. Plastic frames are an exception to this rule: They rest directly on the face, so not much can be done about them rubbing on the patient's cheeks. Some adjustments may need to be done to the frame to make it fit the patient correctly. This is common. A common rule of thumb is that when the patient is wearing the frame, his or her pupils should fall near the center of the frame.

> It is a good idea to fit smaller children in glasses that are a bit too big (not a lot) so that they have growing room. (Children grow quickly and parents do not want to buy new frames and lenses every 6 months.)

4. *Temple length*—The temples need to be the right length to ensure that the glasses stay on and do not pinch. When the temple is fitted behind the ear (by bending around it) it should fit the contour of the ear and the tip should fall approximately two thirds the way down the back of the ear. If the temples are too long, you can cut them to fit or call the manufacturer to see what different lengths are offered for that particular frame.

5. *Bridge size and fit*—It is important that the nosepiece fits correctly for the same reasons it is important that the temples fit correctly: The glasses need to stay on and not pinch. The most important thing to remember is, the bridge of the glasses needs to be wide or narrow enough to allow the nosepieces to contour around the nose as much as possible.

6. *Type of frame*—Most patients have a preference about what type of frame they prefer (e.g., plastic, metal, rimless, drill mount). Rimless and drill-mount frames require more delicate handling. If your patient wants rimless or drill-mount frames, you should warn him or her that these frames are more delicate than other frames because the lenses are exposed, and any pressure applied to the frame is applied directly to the lenses, which could break them. (This means the patient must not sleep in these frames.)

FACE SHAPES

Following are the basic face shapes you will see and some suggested frame styles. When frame styling a patient, you should look at his or her face shape and pick a frame that is opposite the face to balance his or her facial features.

Face Shape		Frame Style
Oval		Square
		Round
		Cat eye
		Octagon
		Oval
		Aviator

Oval is the easiest face shape to fit. Any style will look good.

Round		Square
		Octagon
		Oval

Triangular		Round
		Oval

Reverse triangular	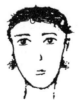	Round
		Cat eye
		Oval

Diamond	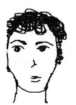	Round
		Oval
		Octagon

FIGURE 3-3 Face shapes.

Continued

Face Shape		Frame Style
Square		Round
		Oval
		Octagon
		Cat eye

FIGURE 3-3 Cont'd

TAKING MEASUREMENTS

Before taking any measurements, you should always adjust the frame to fit the patient comfortably.

REVIEW OF THE TERMS USED WHEN MEASUREMENTS ARE TAKEN

OC Ocular center.

OC Height (OC Ht) Ocular center height.

PD Pupillary distance (e.g., monocular PD, binocular PD)

Segment Height (Seg Ht) When measuring the seg ht, always make sure you are eye level with the patient so that you do not measure too high or too low. When taking measurements, you always measure the PD first. This measurement must be taken for every pair of glasses, no matter what style of lens is chosen. There are two different ways to measure a PD: with a PD ruler or with a pupillometer.

TAKING MEASUREMENTS WITH A PD RULER

1. Make sure that you are standing eye level with the patient. You do not want to stand too high or too low because the eyes tend to pull in more when not gazing directly forward. Thus your measurement will be incorrect.
2. Tell the patient to focus his or her right eye at your left eye.
3. Line up the 0 in the center of the pupil on the patient's right eye. Hold still.
4. Tell the patient to focus his or her left eye on your right eye and locate the center of the pupil. The number on the PD ruler now gives you the binocular PD. If you want to find the monocular PD, measure each eye from the center of the pupil to the center of the bridge of the nose.

Patient is focused on your right eye

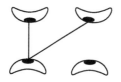

Place PD ruler at 0
in the middle of the pupil

Patient is focused in your left eye

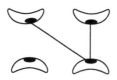

When the patient is focused,
locate the number that
falls in the center of the pupil

FIGURE 3-4 Measuring the pupillary distance (PD).

TAKING THE PD MEASUREMENT WITH A PUPILLOMETER

To use the pupillometer, you must set it on infinity (∞) and ask the patient to look at the light inside. Place the lines directly in the center of the pupils. Move the pupillometer, and you have the measurement. Most pupillometers provide both the mono PD and the binocular PD.

TAKING MEASUREMENTS FOR DIFFERENT LENS STYLES

Single Vision Measurements The following measurements are needed for a single vision lens:

1. PD
2. OC Ht

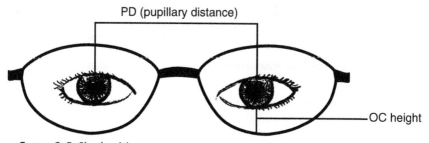

FIGURE 3-5 Single vision measurements.

Lined Bifocal Measurements The following measurements are needed for the ST 28, ST 35, ST 45, and so on:

1. PD
2. OC Ht
3. Seg ht

Remember to measure the seg ht from the lower eyelid to the farthest bottom inside point of the frame. You should use a water marker to make a line where the line would be for the bifocal. Ask the patient to imagine that this is the line for the bifocal. Tell him or her to look around, and explain that the reading area would start directly below the line you have drawn. Ask him or her whether the line is too high, too low, or just right. Make any necessary adjustments to the height of the bifocal to suit the patient. Now is the time to adjust the height of the line, not after the lens has been cut. It may take more time for you to make the sale, but you prevent a remake on the lenses because the measurement was wrong. Making sure the lens is correct the first time saves you and the patient money, time, and aggravation. The minimal segment height for a lined bifocal is approximately 11 to 12 mm. This ensures enough reading area.

> When you are measuring a child for bifocals, you need to measure approximately 2 mm high, because children tend to drop their heads when reading instead of dropping just their eyes.
> People who hold their head high need to be measured lower than normal because they will keep looking through their bifocal when they are looking forward.
> People who hold their head low need to be measured a little higher than normal so that they will use their bifocal.

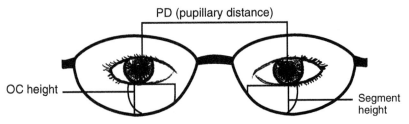

FIGURE 3-6 Lined bifocal measurements.

Lined Trifocal Measurements The following measurements are needed for the 7 × 28, 8 × 35, and so on:

1. PD
2. OC
3. Seg ht

Remember to measure the seg ht from the middle of the iris to the farthest bottom inside point of the frame. Just as you would do for a lined bifocal, mark a line where the line would be to be sure of your measurement. The minimal segment height for a lined trifocal is 18 to 19 mm. This ensures enough reading area.

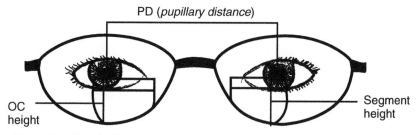

FIGURE 3-7 Lined trifocal measurements.

PAL Measurements The following are measurements needed for any no-line bifocal:

1. Mono PD
2. OC ht (the same as the segment height for the progressive lens)

Measuring the OC height of a PAL is the same as measuring the segment height. It is also acceptable to measure 1 or 2 mm below the center of the pupil. The minimal segment height for most PALs is 19 to 21 mm, depending on the manufacturer. The measurements for progressive lenses are similar to those for single vision lenses. An easy way to be accurate most of the time is to mark the OC height for the progressive lens with a water marker by making a dot (or line) across the pupils. Ask the patient to look around. Then ask him or her whether the dot (or line) is right in, above, or below his or her line of sight. If it is exactly in the middle of his or her vision, you should measure from the dot (or line) to the farthest bottom inside point of the frame. This is the segment height.

If your patient is currently wearing bifocals (lined or no lines), when you measure him or her, it is best to ask whether he or she is comfortable with where the current bifocal line sits. He or she will let you know whether it is too high or too low or whether it feels right. If the old bifocal or trifocal is comfortable, you should try to make sure the new one sits in the same place. Some patients like to wear their bifocal lower or higher than normal. That is all right as long as the patient is comfortable with his or her vision.

LENSOMETER

The *lensometer* is the instrument used to "read" the prescription (or power) of lenses. The lenses may be a semifinished blank that needs to be cut to fit the frames or they may already be mounted in the frame and the prescription needs to be verified. You may also check for prism with a lensometer.

PARTS OF THE LENSOMETER

Power Drum   Identifies the power of the lens. It is located on the right-hand side. Plus power numbers are located above the "0" mark and minus powers are located below the "0" mark. On some lensometers, the plus numbers are written in red and the minus numbers are written in black. The markings for the powers are in 0.12 steps from 0 to 3.00 diopters plus and minus. If the prescription is more than 3.00 diopters plus and minus, the markings are in 0.25 (quarter) steps.

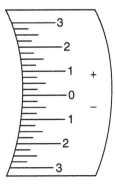

Figure **3-8** Power drum.

Axis Wheel   Identifies the location of the cylinder in degrees. It is located on the back of the lensometer. It is marked in 1-degree steps from 0 to 180 degrees.

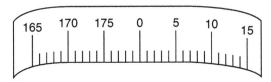

Figure **3-9** Axis wheel.

Eyepiece   The part of the lensometer you look into. It is on the top and is used to focus the image. You must always focus the lensometer for your vision before you "read" any lens.

Prism Ring   Part that allows you to determine the amount and the location of prism. It is located below the eyepiece. This should always be checked before a lens is read to make sure it is set to 0 and that no prism is going to be induced when marking the lens.

Lens Table   The platform on which the lens or the pair of glasses rests while a reading is being taken. It moves up and down.

Lens Holder   A circular piece used to hold the lens in place while taking a reading. If the lens needs to be moved, you should always lift up the lens holder when you are moving the lens. If you do not lift the lens holder, you may scratch the lens.

Lens Stop The circular piece against which the back side of the lens rests. You should always make sure the back side of the lens is on the lens stop when taking a reading.

IMAGES YOU WILL SEE INSIDE THE LENSOMETER

Reticules The "rings" or "bull's eye" that help you center the lens. They are used to measure prism. They will be numbered from the second inside ring, which is number 1, to the outside ring, which is number 4. Each ring represents 1 diopter of prism. The first inside ring represents 1/2 diopter of prism.

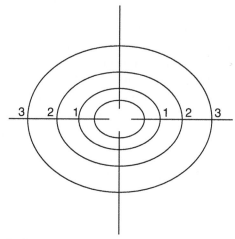

FIGURE 3-10 Reticules.

Meridian lines The lines that represent the power of the lens. The three *thin* lines represent the *sphere power*. The three *thick* lines represent the *cylinder power*.

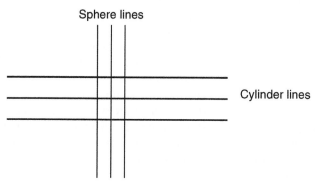

FIGURE 3-11 Meridian lines.

VERIFYING AN UNCUT LENS

1. Turn on the lensometer and focus the eyepiece for your vision. The numbers on the prism ring should be clear.
2. Place the lens on the lens table (right eye first) and secure it against the lens stop with the lens holder.
3. Center the meridian lines on the reticules. Make sure the lines are in the center of the bull's eye. If the lens needs to be moved, you must always pull the lens holder up so that you avoid scratching the lens.
4. Set the power drum to the sphere power that is written.
5. Set the axis wheel to the axis that is written.
6. The thin lines should be clear and straight. If they are not, you should lift the lens holder and turn the lens until the thin lines are clear and straight. (If the lens is spherical, both sets of lines, thin and thick, should be clear at the same time and there is no axis to find.)
7. Move the power drum to the cylinder power and make sure the thick lines are clear and straight. For example, the prescription reads as follows: OD – 2.50 –0.50 × 150. Adding the cylinder power and the spherical power gives you the number on the power drum where the thick lines are clear and straight. In this example, the cylinder power would be –3.00. If the prescription had been +2.50 –0.50 × 150, the cylinder power on the power drum would read +2.00. If the signs are alike (+ and + or – and –), you add the numbers. If the signs are different (+ and –), you subtract the smaller number from the greater number and take the sign of the greater number.
8. Mark the lens with the lens marker. Mark the dots on the back side of the lens with a water marker and write "R" at the top for right eye.
9. Repeat for the lens for the left eye.

VERIFYING GLASSES

1. Turn on the lensometer and focus the eyepiece for your vision. The numbers on the prism ring should be clear.
2. Place the glasses on the lens table (right eye first) and secure them against lens stop with the lens holder.
3. Center the meridian lines in the reticules. Make sure the lines are in the center of the "bull's eye." If the lens needs to be moved, you must always pull the lens holder up so that you avoid scratching the lens.
4. Turn the power drum until the thin lines are clear and the thick lines are fuzzy. If both sets of lines are clear and straight at the same time, the lens is spherical (i.e., it has no cylinder power, no correction for astigmatism).
5. Turn the axis wheel until the thin lines are straight and unbroken in the middle. (Leave the power drum alone when you do this. You are trying to find the location of the axis; you have already found the power.)
6. Record the number on the power drum as your spherical power and the number on the axis wheel as your axis. Make sure you also record whether it is plus or minus.

7. Look back into the lensometer and turn the power drum until the thick lines are clear. If you have found the axis correctly, the thick lines will be straight. You will not touch the axis wheel again.

8. Subtract the number you find for the clear thick lines from the number you recorded for the spherical power; the difference is the cylinder power. (The number you read for the spherical power should always be greater than the number you read for the cylinder power. If it is not, you have read the power 90 degrees off. You can simply transpose the prescription. See Transposing).

9. Repeat for the lens for the left eye.

Spherical power lines are clear and broken

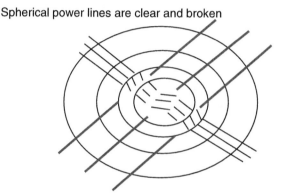

Cylinder lines are blurry and broken

FIGURE 3-12 Broken lines off axis.

Clear, straight spherical power lines mean the spherical power

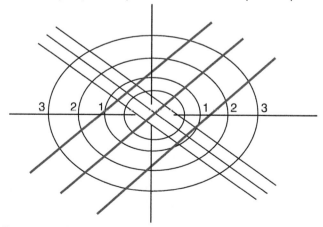

Fuzzy, straight cylinder lines mean the axis is located and the cylinder power still needs to be located

FIGURE 3-13 Straight lines on axis.

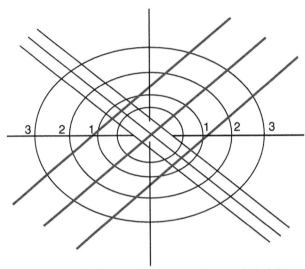

When both sets of lines are clear and straight
at the same time, it indicates, NO cylinder power

FIGURE **3-14** Straight lines spherical lens.

TRANSPOSING

Transposition (transposing) is the way you change the signs of the cylinder from plus to minus (or minus to plus) and keep the power the same.

HOW TO TRANSPOSE A PRESCRIPTION

1. Add the cylinder power to the sphere. When the signs are alike (– and – or + and +), you add the numbers together and keep the same sign for the sphere. When the signs are opposite (– and +), you subtract the smaller number from the larger number and use the sign of the larger number for the sphere. This gives you the new sphere power.
2. Change the sign of the cylinder from plus to minus. Do not change the power, only the sign.
3. Change the axis by 90 degrees. If the axis is less than 90 degrees, add 90 degrees. If the axis is more than 90 degrees, subtract 90 degrees.

For example, if the prescription is –2.75 +0.50 × 90, and you want to put it in minus cylinder form, you would transpose as follows:

$$-2.75 + (+)0.50 = -2.25$$
$$-2.25 -0.50 \times 90$$
$$-2.25 -0.50 \times 180 \; \textit{final answer}$$

You use the same formula to change the cylinder from minus to plus. For example, if the prescription is –2.75 –0.50 × 90, you would transpose as follows:

$$-2.75 + (-)0.50 = -3.25$$
$$-3.25 + 0.50 \times 90$$
$$-3.25 + 0.50 \times 180 \; \textit{final answer}$$

> When you change a bifocal prescription into a single vision, near prescription, that is also called *transposing* the prescription. To make a reading prescription, add the Add power to the *sphere* power only. Do not change the cylinder power or the axis. To make an intermediate prescription, add half the Add power to the sphere power. (Add half the Add power for a trifocal prescription, unless otherwise noted by the doctor.)

The following example shows the calculations to find the reading prescription from a bifocal prescription. If the bifocal prescription is OD –2.75 –0.50 × 180 Add +2.00 OS –3.25 –0.75 × 98, the reading prescription is calculated as follows:

$$-2.75 \; (+) +2.00 = -0.75$$
$$-3.25 \; (+) +2.00 = -1.25$$

The new reading prescription is OD –0.75 –0.50 × 180 OS –1.25 –0.75 × 98.

LEVEL 3 ASSESSMENT

1. Aspheric lenses have:
   A. A single curve on the front and back surfaces
   B. A single curve on the front surface and two curves on the back side
   C. A series of curves on the front surface and one or two curves on the back side
   D. No curves on the front surface and three curves on the back side
2. Unwanted prism is:
   A. Prism in a lens not prescribed by the doctor
   B. Prism in a lens prescribed by the doctor
   C. Prism in a lens going up
   D. Prism in a lens going out
3. Choosing a lens for the patient depends mostly on:
   A. His or her skin tone
   B. The amount of swimming he or she does
   C. The distance between his or her eyes
   D. His or her prescription
4. Which of the following is *not* considered when choosing a lens?
   A. Lens material
   B. Temple length
   C. Type of lens
   D. Light sensitivity
5. True or False: You should try to choose a lens before choosing a frame.
6. Which of the following do *not* make a good combination?
   A. Polycarbonate lens and ARC
   B. High plus lens and aspheric design
   C. High plus lens and rimless frame
   D. High minus lens and polycarbonate
7. True or False: There are six basic face shapes.
8. For an oval face, the best frame is:
   A. A square frame
   B. An octagon frame
   C. Any shape looks good
   D. A round frame
9. List four things to consider when frame styling a patient.
10. True or False: The lifestyle of the patient is a concern when choosing a frame to fit the lenses chosen.
11. If the patient's prescription is for bifocals, this tells you:
    A. Where the patient reads
    B. The minimal depth the frame needs to be
    C. The color the frame should be
    D. The temple length of the frame

12. If the patient plays sports often, the frame should be:
    A. A full frame
    B. A rimless frame
    C. A drill-mount frame
    D. A tinted frame

13. When choosing a good eye size frame for the patient, a good rule of thumb is that the bottom of the eye wire should fall:
    A. Down to the tip of the lower lid
    B. Half way down the contour of the ear
    C. All the way down to the tip of the nose
    D. Half way down the nose

14. The measurements to take for a single vision lens are:
    A. Seg ht and OC ht
    B. PD only
    C. PD and OC
    D. Seg ht and PD

15. A mono PD is:
    A. The height of the bifocal
    B. The height to the pupil
    C. The pupils measured together
    D. The pupils measured separately

16. To what part of the eye is a traditional lined bifocal measured?
    A traditional lined trifocal?
    A progressive addition lens (PAL)?

17. To what part of the frame is the bifocal or trifocal measured?
    A. Inside bottom of frame
    B. Outside bottom of frame
    C. Outside of frame directly below the pupil
    D. Inside of frame directly below the pupil

18. The minimal segment height for a lined bifocal is:
    A. 3-4 mm
    B. 19-20 mm
    C. 15-16 mm
    D. 11-12 mm

19. The part of the lensometer that is used to locate the power of the lens is:
    A. The axis wheel
    B. The power drum
    C. The meridian lines
    D. The eyepiece

20. The meridian lines to locate the axis correctly are:
    A. Straight and clear
    B. Fuzzy and broken
    C. Broken and clear
    D. Fuzzy

21. The meridian lines to locate the sphere are:
    A. Thick
    B. Fuzzy
    C. Thin
    D. Broken
22. To transpose a prescription means to:
    A. Change the axis
    B. Divide the sphere and add it to the cylinder power
    C. Change the signs of the cylinder without changing the power of the lens
    D. Make a distance prescription from a trifocal prescription
23. True or False: You can transpose a prescription to make a reading prescription from a trifocal prescription.
24. When transposing a prescription, you *never* change the:
    A. Spherical power
    B. Cylinder power
    C. Axis
    D. Add power

LEVEL 4

Optician

OBJECTIVES

- Finish your education so that you will be able to fulfill all of the job requirements of an optician.
- Be able to work on your own with little or no assistance.

TASKS TO MASTER

- Filling out **job orders and** making **sales**
- **Dispensing glasses**
- **Dispensing contact lenses**
- **Troubleshooting**
- **Verifying glasses** (being able to use the lensometer competently)

You should have little supervision while performing all of these tasks. Your work should be double-checked until you have mastered this level.

LEVEL 4 SCHEDULE

Congratulations! You now have reached Level 4. In Level 4, you will be learning the final touches to becoming an optician. An assessment will be given to check your progress.

LEVEL 4 OPTICIAN

Task

Stage 1

Read assigned material: *Job Orders and Sales*	
Continue practicing all tasks learned in previous levels	
Start filling out job orders	
Start doing sales from start to finish	

Stage 2

Read assigned material: *Dispensing Glasses*	
Read assigned material: *Dispensing Contact Lenses*	
Continue filling out job orders	
Continue doing sales from start to finish	
Start dispensing glasses and contact lenses	

Stage 3

Read assigned material: *Troubleshooting*	
Continue filling out job orders	
Continue doing sales from start to finish	
Continue dispensing glasses and contact lenses	
Become more involved in troubleshooting a patient's problem	

Stage 4

Read assigned material: *Verifying Glasses*	
Continue filling out job orders	
Continue doing sales from start to finish	
Continue dispensing glasses and contact lenses	
Start verifying glasses for the doctors and patients	

Stage 5

Each stage and each level has gotten you to this point.
Perfect your skills as an optician and you will be ready for
the next step. Your next step should be becoming
certified. Congratulations and good luck in your
future career as an optician.

JOB ORDERS AND SALES

JOB ORDERS

The information you need on every job order does not change. You need to make sure that every order for glasses has the following information, or the glasses will not be made correctly.

INFORMATION NEEDED FOR JOB ORDERS

1. Patient's name
2. Order number or invoice number as a reference
3. Prescription
4. Add power (if bifocal or trifocal)
5. Pupillary distance
6. Segment height (if bifocal or trifocal)
7. Ocular center height
8. Prism (if prescribed)
9. Base curve (if a specific one is needed)
10. Lens material (e.g., polycarbonate)
11. Type of lens desired (e.g., ST 28)
12. Frame measurements (A, B, ED, and DBL)
13. Frame name and manufacturer
14. Any tints or coatings (e.g., antireflective coating [ARC]) that need to be applied (When ordering a tint, you must always indicate the color, the shade [how dark or light], and whether it is solid or gradient.)
15. Any special instructions for the patient (e.g., patient likes to wear bifocal low)
16. What type of frame has been chosen (e.g., metal, rimless, drill mount)

There are many different ways to write an order; however, the laboratory must have all of this information to be able to process the glasses.

SALES

Selling glasses is very different from selling anything else in the retail business. It is a mixed world of retail and medical need. Many choices of frames (colors, styles, name brands) and lenses (thin, tinted, specialty coatings) are available. However, there is the medical need of the patient. He or she needs to have the best vision possible with the available technology and science.

You should always greet the patient with a smile and be ready to help. The patient expects you to be the expert. You should know your products, their benefits, and their drawbacks. You need to start a conversation with the patient to determine his or her needs and wants so that you can fit him or her with the best possible pair of glasses. You should always start with quoting the most premium, top-of-the-line product and work down from there. This is called selling from the *top down*. As discussed in Level 3, it is beneficial to choose the lenses before choosing a frame. The most important thing is for the patient to see well, so choosing the best lens to suit his or her needs and lifestyle, before choosing a frame, is the best way to meet the needs of the patient. The type and style of lens chosen may also narrow down the choice of frames.

Following is a list of questions to ask the patient to determine what type of lens and coatings he or she may need:

1. What will be the main use of the glasses? Reading? Computer work? Playing sports? Driving? Everything from driving to reading?
2. Do you have trouble with driving at night? Reflections from the computer? Reflections from the back of your glasses?
3. Do you have trouble with light sensitivity? Indoors? Outdoors?

The prescription will give you a chance to offer the best lens material available. This is covered in more detail in the sections *Choosing Lenses* and *Frame Styling* in Level 3.

Some offices have a questionnaire for patients to fill out to get the same information. If your office has one, use it. If your office does not have a questionnaire, you can open the conversation with the patient by explaining that you are not trying to pry into his or her life, you are just trying to determine how the lens is going to be used. Tell the patient that with this information, you can meet his or her visual needs and fit his or her lifestyle. If you state this in the beginning, the patient will be more open with you about his or her needs and wants and will not expect you to be a mind reader. Another helpful tip is to always offer ARC, because it is beneficial to the patient's visual acuity.

After the lenses have been chosen, the next step is to pick out a frame. Remember to consider the following factors:

1. Shape of the frame
2. Color of the frame
3. Eye size
4. Temple length
5. Bridge size and fit
6. Type of frame

All of these are covered in detail in the section *Frame Styling* in Level 3.

After the lenses and frame have been chosen, the next step is to take the measurements. The details for this can be found in the section *Taking Measurements* in Level 3. Explain each step to the patient (what you are doing and the purpose it serves). This makes the patient feel like part of the process and puts him or her more at ease with the whole sales process.

Once the measurements have been taken, you should review with the patient each item and its purpose. This review gives the patient the chance to change the order, and it clarifies the order. It gives the power of choice and responsibility to the patient. It ensures that you are being straightforward and that you will inform the patient without pressure. It is also your opportunity to double-check the job order and make sure you did not leave anything out.

Next, you need to collect payment. It is no secret that glasses are expensive. The most effective way to ask for payment is to simply ask the patient how he or she will be paying. Cash? Credit card? Check? You should ask your manager which payment options your store accepts. Therefore if the patient cannot pay in full at the time of the sale, you will be able to give other options.

At the time of payment, you should tell the patient an expected time glasses will be ready. Check with your laboratory or your manager for the turnaround times on all products. It takes longer for some lenses to be returned from the laboratory than it does for others. It is also a good idea to write the date on the patient's copy of the receipt or ticket so that he or she has a reminder of when the glasses will be ready.

Finally, thank the patient for their business and state that you look forward to seeing them again. Remember, even though you did not get personal with the patient, you did establish a relationship with that person through the sales process. You also just took a good bit of money from the patient. Keep the patient happy and he or she will keep you in business.

Following is a summary of the whole sales process:

1. Greet the patient with a smile and be ready to help.
2. Choose the lenses.
3. Choose the frame.
4. Take the necessary measurements.
5. Review in detail what has been chosen.
6. State the cost.
7. Collect payment.
8. Inform the patient of the date the glasses should be ready.
9. Thank the patient for his or her business.

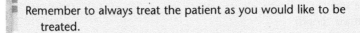
Remember to always treat the patient as you would like to be treated.

DISPENSING GLASSES

Following is what you need to do when the patient comes back to pick up his or her glasses. You will adopt your own way of presenting these things.

1. Verify patient name and address when the patient comes in to pick up his or her glasses. If you have two patients with the same name, this helps avoid confusion.
2. Always tell the patient to wet the lenses before wiping them, because dust settles on the lenses and wiping them dry could scratch the lenses.

3. Tell the patient that he or she should *not* fall asleep with the glasses on, because this could damage the frame and break the lenses.
4. If the patient has transition lenses, make sure he or she knows that it takes a few days for the lenses to fully activate.
5. If the lenses have an ARC, remind the patient to wipe the lens lightly (*not* hard). The lighter you wipe, the cleaner the lens gets. The harder you wipe, the more it will smear.
6. Always make sure the patient's vision with the glasses is good before he or she leaves. If the patient has bifocals or trifocals, make sure you give him or her something to read in addition to having him or her look around.
7. Always make necessary adjustments when the patient picks up his or her glasses. The glasses may lose some alignment after going through the laboratory.
8. If the patient is wearing a progressive lens for the first time, instruct him or her again on how to point his or her nose at anything he or she wants to see. Instruct the patient to pick out something to look at and move his or her head up and down, to note the change in vision. There will also be distortion in the patient's peripheral vision because of the lens design. He or she will have to learn where to focus to get the best vision, depending on how far away the object is. Progressive lenses have no lines to tell the patient where the prescription changes. Tell the patient that it may take at least 2 weeks to adjust to the new lenses, especially if the prescription has changed.
9. Always end the dispensing by telling the patient, "Let us know if there is anything more we can do to help you with your new glasses and how well you are doing with them." *Never* imply that the patient may have problems by saying, "If you have any problems give us a call." This will leave the patient with the impression that you anticipate problems for him or her.
10. If there is a balance due on the order, make sure you collect before the patient leaves.
11. After the patient has picked up his or her glasses and you have completed all necessary paperwork, you need to document on the job order the date, what was done, and your initials (e.g., Dispensed 11-15-02 DW).

DISPENSING CONTACT LENSES

You may not be asked to dispense contact lenses in some offices, but in most cases you will. Following is what you need to do when dispensing contact lenses:

1. Verify patient name and address when the patient comes in to pick up the contact lenses. If you have two patients with the same name, this helps avoid confusion.

2. Verify that the contact lenses (in vials or packs) match what was ordered on the job order.

3. Make sure the vials or packs are marked right and left for the appropriate prescription.

4. Make sure the patient has cleaning solutions. These may have been given to the patient at the time of his or her examination. You should ask the patient if he or she needs more solutions at this time. It also reminds the patient to clean the contact lenses.

5. If there are any special instructions, make sure that you follow them (e.g., the doctor would like to see the patient with the contact lenses on when the patient picks up the lenses).

6. Depending on the store where you work, you may have to teach the patient how to insert and remove the contact lenses. You will also have to teach the patient how to clean and care for the contact lenses. This is usually done at the time of the examination, but in some cases the patient has to wait until the contact lenses are ordered and have arrived. As stated before, this is usually the duty of the doctor's technician, but you may be called on to do it. Ask your trainer if this applies to you.

7. If there is a balance due on the order, make sure you collect before the patient leaves.

8. After the patient has picked up his or her contact lenses and you have completed all necessary paperwork, you need to document on the job order the date, what was done, and your initials (e.g., Dispensed 11-15-02 DW).

TROUBLESHOOTING

You will practice troubleshooting when a patient's prescription is bothering him or her. Based on the patient's complaints and your findings, you can determine whether the lenses have a defect or the patient needs a new prescription. When a patient makes any complaint about his or her lenses and prescription, you should do the following:

1. Listen closely to what the patient is telling you and repeat it back to make sure you understand exactly what is going on. Ask questions such as the following:
   A. How long has this been going on?
   B. Is the problem in only one eye?
   C. Is it only when you read or only when you look out far away?
   These types of questions narrow down the problem.

2. Double-check all measurements to make sure the lenses were made to the measurements taken.

3. Double-check the prescription to make sure it was made to what the doctor ordered.

4. Make sure the frame is sitting on the patient correctly.
5. Check with the laboratory if the measurements are wrong; new lenses will have to be made. If the optician took or wrote down the wrong measurements, new lenses will have to be made.
6. If all the measurements are correct and you have adjusted the frame to accommodate and the patient is still not seeing well, the doctor will have to see the patient again and there may be a change in the prescription. New lenses will have to be made.

Following are some common patient complaints you might hear.

Complaint "My eyes are pulling."
Could Be Unwanted prism resulting from the optical centers being in the wrong place. This occurs when the patient feels the pulling sensation to the right, to the left, up, or down. If the pulling sensation is straight ahead, as though the eyes are coming out of the sockets, the prescription may be too strong.

Complaint "My vision is blurry. Things are not clear or crisp. I'm having trouble seeing."
Could Be

1. The lenses are made to the wrong power or the axis is wrong.
2. The prescription given by the doctor is wrong.
3. The patient has developed an eye disease.
4. It is time for a new eye examination.
5. The glasses need adjusting. In this situation, consider every possibility.

Complaint "I have to hold my head up too high to see through the bifocal [trifocal]."
Could Be The bifocal or trifocal is made too low. Check the measurements.

Complaint "I have to turn my head to read with my invisible bifocal."
Could Be The placement of the optical centers is wrong. Check the measurements.

Complaint "Things seem to curve when I look at them."
Could Be The lenses are not sitting at the correct angle on the face. Check the difference between the old base curve and the new base curve. In addition, check the axis. Patients wearing glasses for the first time may experience a "fish bowl" effect for the first few days because of never having lenses before.

Complaint "I have to put my head down to see things far away."
Could Be The bifocal is made too high. Check the measurements.

VERIFYING GLASSES

Following are the things you as a dispenser need to verify on a pair of glasses. This is also called *checking out* or *neutralizing* a pair of glasses.

1. Power of the lens. If the lens is single vision, there is only one power to check. If the lens is a bifocal or trifocal, check the distance and the near prescriptions.
2. PD measurement. If the glasses are bifocals or trifocals, check the distant and near PD.
3. Prism. If the PD or OC is not ground correctly (not sitting right over the pupils), check for horizontal and vertical prism.
4. Segment height on bifocals, trifocals, and PAL.
5. Ocular center height for all lenses.
6. Base curves (front only).
7. Coatings (e.g., tints, UV, ARC, transition). Make sure any coatings are correct.
8. Scratches, scuffs, and/or chips. Verify that glasses are free of blemishes.
9. Waves in the lens. (Distortion in the lens looks like a wave in the prescription.) There will always be distortion on the outer edge (peripheral) if the lens is a PAL or a high prescription.
10. Defects in coloration. Discoloration really shows on darker tints.
11. Frame alignment. The frame should look straight. The temples should not bend out nor should they be twisted. The nose pads should also be straight and not bent or twisted. If the frames are out of alignment, the patient's vision could be directly affected.

When you are verifying the glasses, remember that they can be "off" by a certain amount and the patient's vision should not be affected. Every laboratory adheres to tolerance standards that are published by the American National Standards Institute and the Opticians Association of America. These standards are otherwise known as *ANSI standards Z80.1–1999*.

Following is a list of the basic standards. The ANSI standards Z80.1 is a more detailed list.

Power Tolerance		Allowed To Be Off
Sphere power	0.00 to ±6.50D	±0.13D
	Above ±6.50D	2% of the power
Cylinder power	0.00 to ±2.00D	±0.13D
	2.13 to ±4.50D	±0.25D
	Above ±4.50D	4% of the power

Add power	If distance power is	
	Plano to ±8.00D	±0.13D
	Above ±8.00D	±0.25D
AXIS		
	0.12 to 0.50	7 degrees
	0.50 to 0.75	5 degrees
	0.75 to 1.50	3 degrees
	1.50 and above	2 degrees

Prism Power One-third prism diopter is allowed to be induced to prescription in any direction.

Segment Placement Allowed to be off by 1 mm in height and 2.5 mm in the distance apart from each other (near PD).

Thickness Allowed to be off by 0.3 mm of what is specified.

Waves Allowed to be off by 1.00D (does not apply within 6 mm of edge of the eye wire).

Base Curve Allowed to be off by ±0.75D of what is specified.

LEVEL 4 ASSESSMENT

1. What information is *not* needed on a job order?
   A. Patient's name
   B. Cost of the lenses from the laboratory
   C. Prescription
   D. Frame measurements
2. True or False: It is important to know what type of frame the patient has to get the best lens possible.
3. When making a sale, it is important to:
   A. Set an appointment to get measurements taken
   B. Clean the patient's old glasses before taking measurements
   C. Reassure the patient and inform him or her of every move
   D. Give the option to pay in full at pickup
4. What is the first thing you should do in the selling process?
   A. Collect payment for the glasses
   B. Take the measurements
   C. Explain the job order
   D. Choose the lenses
5. When you are dispensing glasses, it is important to make sure the patient knows:
   A. How to use the lenses he or she has just bought
   B. Who to ask for a refund
   C. What brand name the frame is
   D. What problems he or she may encounter
6. When the patient cleans his or her glasses, he or she should:
   A. Know his or her address and phone number
   B. Fall asleep in them
   C. Adjust the frame
   D. Always wet the lens before wiping
7. If the patient has purchased bifocals, make sure:
   A. He or she knows how to adjust his or her own glasses
   B. He or she knows how to use the lenses for reading and distance
   C. He or she has paid in full before leaving
   D. He or she know there may be problems
8. True or False: When dispensing a pair of invisible bifocals to a patient who is wearing them for the first time, you should instruct the patient again on how to use the lens.
9. Two things to verifying when dispensing contact lenses are:
   A. The patient's glasses are good and there are no markings on them
   B. The boxes/vials are marked right and left and the type of contact is correct
   C. The patient has enough money to pay and his or her credit is good
   D. The patient has an appointment and has insurance

10. True or False: The doctor is the only person allowed to dispense contact lenses.

11. When you are dispensing contact lenses, make sure the patient has, in addition to the lenses:
    A. An appointment for an examination
    B. Cleaning solutions
    C. A carrying case
    D. Good insurance

12. True or False: The patient should *never* be taught insertion and removal when picking up his or her contact lenses.

13. If the patient has to hold his or her head up to look out of the bifocal, you should:
    A. Loosen the temples
    B. Give more facial wrap to the frame
    C. Loosen the nose pads
    D. Bend the temples down and pull the nose pads in

14. If the patient is seeing reflections on the lens and his or her peripheral vision is distorted, you should:
    A. Loosen the temples
    B. Increase the facial wrap
    C. Loosen the nose pads
    D. Tighten the temples

15. If there is unwanted prism in a patient's glasses, his or her complaint would be:
    A. "I have to look up to read."
    B. "I see reflections on the front of my glasses."
    C. "I see waves."
    D. "My eyes are pulling."

16. When a patient makes a complaint about his or her glasses, you should:
    A. Repeat back to the patient what he or she has told you
    B. Refer the patient to someone else
    C. Schedule an appointment with the doctor
    D. Make sure the frame is the correct color

17. True or False: Checking the frame alignment is not necessary when verifying glasses.

18. List six things to check when verifying glasses.

19. How many degrees off axis is a lens with a −1.25 cylinder allowed to be?
    A. 10
    B. 7
    C. 3
    D. 1

20. A distortion in the lens means:
    A. There are too many scratches on the lens
    B. The base curve is off
    C. There are waves in the lens
    D. The tint is not dark enough

ANSWERS TO ASSESSMENTS LEVELS 1-4

LEVEL 1 ASSESSMENT

1. True
2. B
3. D
4. True
5. B
6. D
7. A
8. C
9. C
10. False
11. B
12. B
13. Surfacing and finishing
14. B
15. D
16. False
17. True
18. D
19. D
20. False

LEVEL 2 ASSESSMENT

1. True
2. C
3. A
4. C
5. B
6. B
7. B
8. A

9. C
10. C
11. B
12. A
13. D
14. True
15. C
16. D
17. A
18. D
19. B
20. C
21. Single vision, bifocal, trifocal, progressive addition lens (PAL)
22. Plastic, glass, polycarbonate, high index
23. B
24. C
25. A
26. C
27. A
28. D
29. True
30. B

LEVEL 3 ASSESSMENT

1. C
2. A
3. D
4. B
5. True
6. C
7. True
8. C
9. Frame shape, color, eye size, temple length, bridge fit, type of frame
10. True
11. B
12. A
13. C
14. C
15. D
16. Lower lid
    Middle of iris
    Middle of pupil
17. A

18. D
19. B
20. A
21. C
22. C
23. True
24. B

LEVEL 4 ASSESSMENT

1. B
2. False
3. C
4. D
5. A
6. D
7. B
8. True
9. B
10. False
11. B
12. False
13. D
14. B
15. D
16. A
17. False
18. Prescription, pupillary distance (PD), prism, segment height, ocular height, base curves, coatings, scratches, waves, defects, frame alignment
19. C
20. C

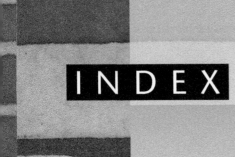

INDEX

O

P

Printed and bound by CPI Group (UK) Ltd, Croydon, CR0 4YY

03/10/2024

01040848-0010